EVANSTON PUBLIC LIBRARY
P9-CSB-020

The Continuum Counseling Series

Language Learning Disabilities

A New and Practical Approach for Those Who Work with Children and Their Families

Sophie L. Lovinger, Mary Ellen Brandell, and Linda Seestedt-Stanford

Foreword by William Van Ornum

Continuum | *New York*

1991

The Continuum Publishing Company
370 Lexington Avenue
New York, NY 10017

Printed in the United States of America

Library of Congress Cataloging-in-Publication Data

Lovinger, Sophie L.
Language learning disabilities : a new and practical approach for those who work with children and their families / Sophie Lovinger, Mary Ellen Brandell, and Linda Seestedt-Stanford ; foreword by William Van Ornum.
p. cm. — (The Continuum counseling series)
Includes bibliographical references.
ISBN 0-8264-0530-4 (cloth)
1. Learning disabilities—United States. 2. Language disorders in children—United States. I. Brandell, Mary Ellen. II. Seestedt-Stanford, Linda. III. Title. IV. Series.
LC4705.L68 1991
371.9—dc20 90-26001
CIP

Contents

Foreword

The Continuum Counseling Series—the first of its kind for a wide audience—presents books for everyone interested in counseling, bringing to readers practical counseling handbooks that include real-life approaches from current research. The topics deal with issues that are of concern to each of us, our families, friends, acquaintances, or colleagues at work.

General readers, parents, teachers, social workers, psychologists, school counselors, nurses and doctors, pastors, and others in helping fields too numerous to mention will welcome these guidebooks that combine the best professional learnings and common sense, written by practicing counselors with expertise in their specialty.

Increased understanding of ourselves and others is a primary goal of these books—and greater empathy is the quality that all professionals agree is essential to effective counseling. Each book offers practical suggestions on how to "talk with" others about the theme of the book, be this in an informal and spontaneous conversation or a more formal counseling session.

Professional therapists will value these books also, because each volume in The Continuum Counseling Series develops its subject in a unified way, unlike many other books that may be either too technical or, as edited collections of papers, may come across to readers as being disjointed. In recent years both the American Psychological Association and the American Psychiatric Association have endorsed books that build on the scientific traditions of each profession but are communicated in an interesting way to general readers. We hope that professors and students in fields such as psychology, social work, psychiatry, guidance and counseling, and other helping fields will find these books to be helpful companion readings for undergraduate and graduate courses.

From nonprofessional counselors to professional therapists, from students of psychology to interested lay readers, The Continuum Counseling Series endeavors to provide informative, interesting, and useful tools for everyone who cares about learning and dealing more effectively with these universal, human concerns.

Language Learning Disabilities

The question and concept of learning disabilities is of great importance to parents and everyone who works with children. An inability to learn academic material in school can have serious emotional and vocational implications for a child, in school and during the years beyond. Now we have a book that addresses learning disabilities in the language-learning sphere. Written by a team of authors representing the disciplines of psychology, audiology, and speech pathology, this book provides a comprehensive framework for understanding language learning disabilities and helping those who struggle with them.

The book provides information on auditory and speech and language development. The authors complement this discussion by looking at how children grown in cognitive and emotional ways. They understand that frustration occurs when children cannot express themselves freely through words and writing. In fact, behavioral and emotional problems, and even juvenile delinquency, have been linked with learning disabilities.

An important part of the book concerns identifying children who possess language-learning disabilities. Since parents and teachers are usually the first ones to notice a potential difficulty, a detailed checklist is provided in order to assist in these assessments. The authors realize that identification of these problems is not an end in itself, but is in reality only the beginning: next, an individualized program must be developed that will not only recognize the problems but accentuate the strengths of each individual child.

Beyond providing a comprehensive presentation in the areas noted, the authors have included very helpful sections on practical suggestions for parents, ideas for the school, and a list of guidelines for the classroom management of children with auditory processing deficits. A glossary includes terms that might be known to specialists but that might help all those who work with these children.

Language Learning Disabilities offers readers important information on a problem that keeps many children and adolescents from functioning to their potential in school and in nonacademic situations. By providing readers not only with a theoretical background on learning disabilities but with numerous practical suggestions as well, the book equips parents, teachers, and counselors to help children whose lives are frustrated by learning disabilities.

William Van Ornum, Ph.D.
Marist College
Poughkeepsie, New York

General Editor
The Continuum Counseling Series

Authors' Note

The identities of the people written about in this book have been carefully disguised in accordance with professional standards of confidentiality and in keeping with their rights to privileged communication with the authors.

Introduction

The three authors of this book, from the disciplines of speech-language pathology, audiology, and clinical child psychology have worked together for approximately twenty years. During this time they have evaluated and developed remediation programs for a vast number of children who have been labeled learning disabled and hyperactive. Consistently they have found these children to be handicapped by central auditory processing problems, language disorders, and emotional and social difficulties. Further, each of them alone, has not been able to effect a resolution of the problems, but working together, from their different disciplines, they have been far more effective in helping these children resolve their problems. The result of their years of collaboration have resulted in this book. Surprisingly, their approach is new and novel, even in this day and age of a team approach because they have cross-fertilized their thinking with each other's discipline creating a coherent approach to the learning disabled child whom they label as Language-Learning Disabled.

Chapters 1 through 3 provide the reader with an overview of audiologic, speech-language, cognitive, and emotional development. Chapter 4 describes the assessment processes to determine the strengths and weaknesses a child may be experiencing in each of the four areas. The fifth chapter deals in depth with remediation strategies and techniques while the sixth chapter attempts to deal with the issues these language-learning disabled youngsters present to their families.

Our frustrations with symptomatic treatment of the presenting problem(s) while ignoring underlying issues has often lead to misdiagnosis. The faddishness of diagnosis based only upon symptomatology or what is au courant has been a primary motivating factor in the development of this book. There are other factors of importance for the authors as well. These include:

1. Narrowness of the focus of each discipline, i.e., looking at a circumscribed area of functioning of a child and not the whole person.
2. Circumscribed area of the professional literature that leads to narrowness rather than breadth of understanding.
3. Differing terminology used for the same syndrome by the different professions that deal with the problems.
4. Treatment that focused upon the small area dealt with by a particular profession, rather than dealing with the wide range of functioning of the child.

The authors firmly feel that the child, or any human being, for that matter, is an integrated whole and must be treated with knowledge of all the parts working as a totality. Pulling the child apart to assess different functions is an artifact that will not be found either in the clinical situation or in the child's day-to-day functioning. We have emphasized clinical observation supported by clinical case material to clarify the issues we have been dealing with for a number of years and to share our understandings with parents, teachers and other professionals who are invested in and concerned with the growth of children cognitively, linguistically, socially, and emotionally.

Our professional discussions made the writing of this book a slow, arduous process. As we moved from our professional orientations, with their specialized languages, clearing up the confusions of the same and similar words used in differing ways, we found that our ideas were similar, complemented each other and enhanced each other's understanding of the problems with which we were dealing. Towards that end we must give special thanks to our very patient and understanding editor, Dr. William Van Ornum. We also give our heartfelt appreciation to our husbands and families who waited as we struggled with the issues we have so far described. Not least of all, our deep appreciation to our secretary, Cheryl Rodden, who could tell us that our manuscript was not reading well because she could not get up to speed in typing.

1

Auditory Development

Stop for a moment and listen. What do you hear? Birds singing, the television in the next room, hammering outside, the teapot boiling, cars passing. The list could go on and on as we are constantly bombarded by sounds, all having varying pitch, loudness level, duration, and sequence. Yet each sound has meaning to us. How did we learn to discriminate these sound differences, associate sound to experience, and then give them meaning? How did we learn to understand sound, to form words to communicate?

The role of the ear in the normal course of speech development cannot be overemphasized. The ear serves as the main feedback mechanism in the development and production of speech. Sound is received by the ear, is interpreted by the brain and a reaction is expressed by use of words. Input of sound to the brain for storage, analysis, and association is done through the ear. Not to hear the human voice is not to develop the ability to speak. It is well established that individuals born with significant hearing loss are unable to develop oral communication naturally. Whereas normal hearing children learn language first, later applying rules, deaf children learn the rules of language first in order for linguistic competencies to be obtained.

Current research is suggesting that even children with hearing loss in one ear, the unilaterally impaired, suffer setbacks in language and thus learning and academic achievement.[1,2,3] Further, it is suggested that children with fluctuating hearing loss due to middle ear infections suffer irreversible disorders in auditory processing, language and learning.[4,5,6,7] Any disruption in the normal reception of sound can impact on a child's total development.

Physiology of Hearing

Hearing is a highly complex activity, employing a complicated neuronal system that is not yet fully describable. The mechanisms of hearing on the peripheral level, in the ear itself, are by far more understood than how the central nervous system (the brain) processes, or gives meaning to the "sound." We do not hear at the level of the ear, but rather in the brain. The ear is the mechanism that transports sounds to the brain for analysis.

In order to understand the theoretical models that follow, and the terminology used throughout the ensuing chapters, a brief explanation of how we hear is necessary. The outer ear, (section 1 on the illustration below), is comprised of the auricle or pinna, and the ear canal. These structures act to accept sound and funnel them into the ear. Cupping your hand to the outer ear is a natural gesture used when we can't hear something. This common practice amplifies sounds by funneling them more directly into the ear canal. In fact, ear trumpets, extensions of the pinna, were man's first hearing aids.

At the end of the ear canal lies the eardrum or tympanic membrane. Attached to this elastic structure is a tiny bone, or ossicle, called the malleus. Through a series of tendons and articulating processes the malleus attaches to the incus, another tiny bone, and the incus to the stapes. These bones, also referred to as the hammer, anvil, and stirrup because of their likeness to these objects, along with the ear drum, form the middle-ear. Section 2 in the illustration above represents the middle ear area. In addition to the eardrum and three bones another important structure called the teustachian tube is present in the middle ear area. This structure brings air into the middle ear from the nose and mouth or the nasopharynx and acts to equalize the pressure outside the head with inside the head. When your "ears pop" that is the eustachian tube opening to allow air in.

The function of the middle ear is to conduct sound through to

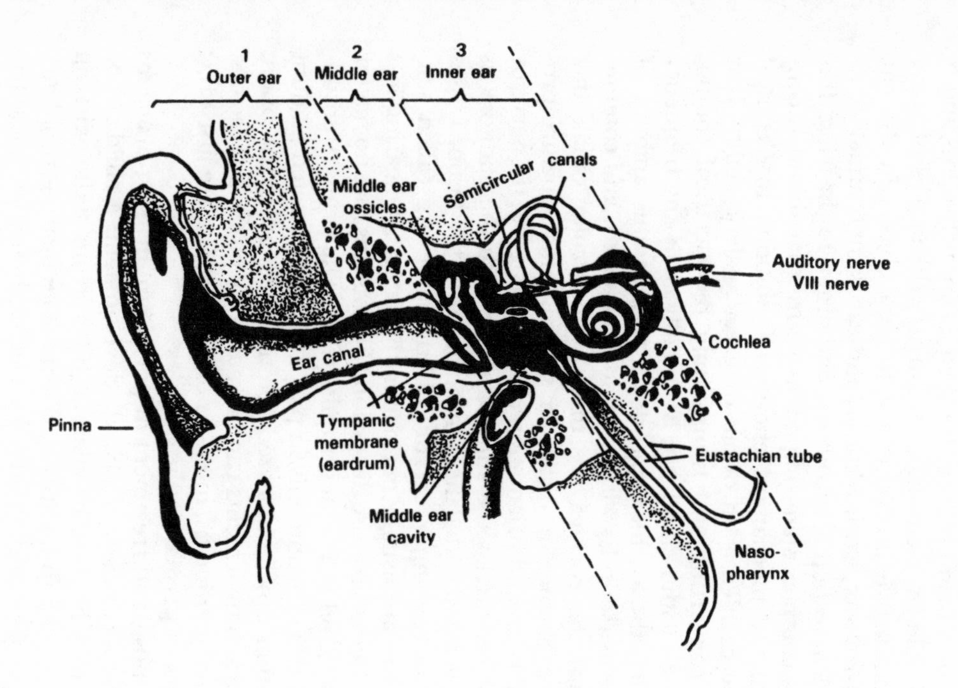

Figure 1-1 Anatomy of the Human Ear.

the inner ear or cochlea. A mechanical vibration of the ossicle causes sound to be "pushed" through to the inner ear. A hearing loss in the outer or middle ear is called a conductive loss and is usually treatable by medication or surgery. Examples of some common conductive problems are foreign objects in the ear canal, excessive wax, ear infections, and eardrum trauma.

The cochlea, section 3, is truly the end organ for hearing. It is here in this complex snail-shaped structure that sound is converted from the mechanical energy of vibration to electrical energy. The cochlea is an organ of great analytic ability. It is capable of converting and transmitting the electrical components of sound with real fidelity. By initially analyzing frequency and intensity, the cochlea encodes a tremendous amount of acoustic events (sounds) with precision. Attached, and communicating with the cochlea are three semi-circular canals that comprise the balance or vestibular system. This structure provides equilibrium and orientation in space. The VIIIth nerve or auditory nerve, carries the stimulation of both the auditory as well as the vestibular (balance) mechanism to the brain. Losses that occur in the inner ear or VIIIth nerve are called sensorineural and are usually permanent in nature. A hearing loss in this area causes acoustic distortion. This means that no matter how loud a sound is, it is never quite clear. The primary encoding process can function only in part and only a limited amount of information can be analyzed for transmission to the brain. Sensorineural impairments can be caused by numerous factors. Birth trauma, meningitis, intense noise, and aging are just a few of the causes of permanent hearing loss.

The diagnosis and treatment of peripheral hearing problems is critical to every aspect of a child's development. A child can be evaluated for a hearing problem at birth by an audiologist, an individual trained to identify and remediate hearing problems. Brainstem-evoked audiometry, an electrophysiologic measurement of sound via monitoring of the brainstem by electrodes, coupled with behavioral observation are effective in identifying hearing problems in the infant. Medication or surgical intervention are helpful in very few cases, and are usually not indicated. A hearing aid is almost always recommended depending on the severity of the loss.

The effects of hearing loss on language and speech depend on the type and severity of the loss, and age at acquisition. Early identification, intervention, and subsequent remediation of a hearing problem in children is critical to optimal speech and language development.

Physiologically the mechanics of the human ear are well understood, but the processing that occurs in the brain for language use is still a mysterious and unanswered area. Illustration 2 represents a very simplified schematic representation of the highly complex central auditory nervous system. From the VIIIth nerve, fibers travel to an area called the cochlear nucleus in the brainstem. The cochlear nucleus is located on each side of the region of the medulla. Research has suggested that this is the initial stage of central auditory processing of sound; that is, a sorting and integrating function for sound occurs at this level. Fibers continue to progress to the region in the temporal lobe of the cortex, called Herschl's Gyrus. The left temporal lobe is involved in the understanding and production of language. It is at this point that knowledge of intracortical connections become limited.

Linguistic competence requires the interaction of several areas of the brain. Sound is heard in one area of the brain, understood in another, and if it is to be spoken must be transmitted to yet another area. The "cooperation" of all these areas are necessary for the reception and accurate use of sound for communication. These association centers are connected to each other and also with centers in the occipital lobe (visual center) that process written language. Problems that occur in the brainstem and brain itself that affect the analysis of sound are called Central Auditory Processing (CAP) problems.

The central auditory processing system, as noted earlier, is an extremely complicated and difficult system to describe as it interacts with so many other processes within the brain and contributes to normal psychological, speech, and language development. Yet it is this higher-level process of listening that we have the least amount of information about. Physiologically, we understand the mechanics of the human ear, but as noted earlier the processing that occurs in the brain for language use is still an area not fully understood by clinicians and researchers alike. Later in this chapter more specific discussion of central auditory processing will be presented.

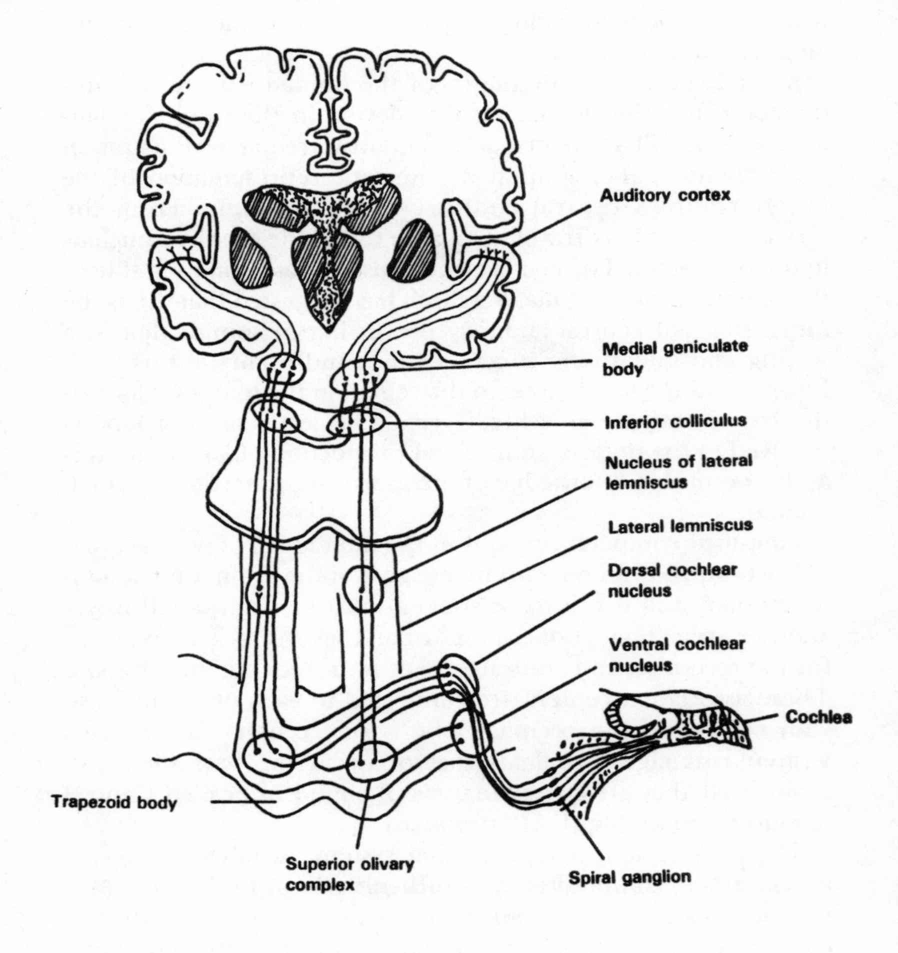

Figure 1-2 Central Auditory Pathways.

Development of Auditory Behavior

In addition to understanding the physiological basis of hearing it is important to be aware of how hearing is integrated into the total development of a child. The development of auditory behavior is hierarchical and closely tied to physical development. Mapping auditory development is dependent on observing an infant's behavioral responses.

It is well established that infants are capable of hearing in utero. By the fifth month of gestation, the hearing mechanism is fully intact. Infants not only hear at birth and react to sounds, but can discriminate sounds on the basis of numerous acoustic variables including bandwidth, duration, rate, pitch, repetition, and loudness.[8,9]

Initially, newborns respond to sounds in a reflexive, almost protective manner. When a loud sound is produced and the infant is in a quiet-awake or light sleep state, a moro reflex or whole body response may be seen. This reflex diminishes after one month of age and eye-widening behavior becomes dominant in response to sounds. At eight weeks of age an infant is no longer disturbed by loud sounds;[10] presumably she/he has begun to learn what is important to respond to in the environment.[11] The infant will still, however, startle to uncommon noises.[12] Occasionally, parents voice concern regarding their newborn's lack of response to loud noises. They report that the infant sleeps through loud stereo music, noisy siblings, the vacuum cleaner, etc. Of course any concern such as this should be followed up with a complete hearing assessment. However, evaluation of the child's noise environment should also be done. If a child lives in a high noise situation, for survival sake his/her system may have adjusted to environmental noise to allow for sleep.

By eight to twelve weeks of age, an infant begins to attune to the human voice, he/she has begun to discriminate and direct his/her attention to sound. It is also at this time that an infant begins to smile in response to a parent's voice and facial expressions. At four months, head movements are beginning to emerge as the infant explores his/her auditory world. Further, the infant responds to stimuli with varying facial expressions. A normally developing infant might be expected to show fifteen different responses to sound at this age.[13] At five months an infant will roll his eyes and then move his head toward a sound source. At six months of age head-turning responses are very marked in infants. Localization to a sound source is a developmental milestone and occurs in 100 percent of normal healthy babies by seven months.[14] Refinement of localization skills to various planes, and response to softer sounds are seen in the infant from eight to twelve months of age.

As noted above, an infant develops more complex but dependable-behaviors in response to sounds as she/he matures. In addition to the overt behavioral awareness of sounds, researchers tell us that infants not only hear and react to sound but appear to respond differentially to various signals,[15,16,9,17] suggesting that at a very early age we learn to associate sound with meaning. Specific repeatable behavioral changes associated with sounds have been noted in the newborn. Low-frequency sounds have been found to act as soothers to infants,[16,9] whereas, high-frequency sounds cause distress. This same tendency is evident in the kinds of signals adults find distressing, such as sirens, phones ringing, or alarms sounding.[15] Has the newborn infant associated meaning to sound? Memory for the low frequency womb sounds the newborn listened to for many months may have conveyed security to the infant and thus low-frequency environmental sounds may also carry the same meaning. Additionally, the research has shown that infants develop the ability to perceive the pitches in the human voice before awareness of other sounds develop. Gesell and Armatruda[10] discuss the observation that basic to the development of an infant is her/his susceptibility to the sound of a voice. Infants respond differently to signals in the primary range for speech. These specific sounds appear to be more effective in eliciting behavioral changes in infants. Later research indicated that an infant will respond to her/his mother's voice to the exclusion of all other stimuli.[13]

In the first year of life much of the infant's active mind is concerned with a readiness to listen. During this preparatory period numerous sound events and their meanings are integrated and related to the other senses. For example, the sound of a spoon in a cup may stimulate an infant to cry for food because she/he has associated that sound with another sensory area, that is, taste. What an infant perceives through audition becomes a part of her/him, is integrated into memory, and thus becomes a building block for language. Early auditory experiences provide a basis for oral language. A feedback mechanism is set up making it possible for a child to accept and analyze incoming and outgoing messages, learn language, and then move among different levels of reference to develop higher level language skills.

Central Auditory Processing

When the peripheral hearing system is normal, but a child has difficulty correctly processing spoken language and other meaningful sounds in his or her environment, central auditory processing problems are suspect. Central auditory integrity is basic to learning. It is a vital factor in speech perception, language development, and cognition. The term Central Auditory Processing encompasses a number of more specific learning difficulties that may appear alone or in combination with other auditory processing problems. Because of the interdependent nature of specific auditory processing skills, a deficit in one area may effect all areas thus impacting on language and learning. These interdependent functions with their combined effects are difficult to isolate as specific clinical entities.

Numerous authors have identified what they have felt to be the salient elements of audition. A listing of those terms are presented in Table 1. Depending on the "model" of auditory processing a particular author utilizes, definitions may differ for the same term. Inconsistencies in the use of these terms only adds to the confusion when defining a "particular" processing area, and thus a child's problem.

Defining these auditory processes more specifically and their related language problems will aid the reader in understanding the complicated, simultaneous relationships that exist. It is apparent from the descriptors below and the examples that follow, that the process of audition is hierarchical; i.e., simple processes are the bases for more complex functioning.

Auditory Attention

Auditory attention involves the ability to attend directly to a particular stimulus, so that what is heard can be transmitted to the brain. Basic localization to a sound and awareness of sound/speech in the environment is important to the development of higher-level tasks. If a child is unable to attend to sound/speech it is obvious that she/he will not be able to discriminate differences between sounds, retain memory for sounds, utilize closure and association skills and analytic ability. A deficit at this basic level will significantly impact on all other audition/language functions. An auditory attention problem may be a consistent problem in a child or may involve isolated periods of inattentiveness when a child is "distracted" from a learning task. The inability to maintain auditory vigilance for a specific period of time affects language and learning significantly. The child suffers "blank spots" in his reception of sound/speech causing educational lags and possibly behavioral problems. This problem is often referred to as Attention Deficit Disorder (ADHD) with or without Hyperactivity. (A more specific discussion of this diagnostic category is presented on page 29.)

Auditory Discrimination

If a child can direct attention to sounds but is unable to determine the differences or similarities between the sounds, difficulties in associating sound with meaning, both for speech and environmental signals may occur. Reading and spelling problems will be the result of problems in this area of auditory behavior. A child may not be able to "hear" the difference between "red" and "bed" or discriminate differences in household sounds like the microwave alarm and the phone ringing. Inability to discriminate between sounds will impact on a child's ability to associate sounds and integrate sound meaning into memory.

Difficulty in reading may occur since the child may have problems discriminating between the beginning, middle, and ending of a word. She/he may have trouble comparing it with the sound of the corresponding parts of other words. Research indicates that the greatest deficit areas in reading are initial consonant sounds, final consonant sounds, and long and short vowel sounds.[18] The phonetic approach to reading is hard for the child with auditory discrimination deficits. He or she may

TABLE 1

Terms identified in literature as being essential elements of audition:

Auditory Association	Auditory Attention
Auditory Analysis	Auditory Blending
Auditory Closure	Auditory Cognition
Auditory Comprehension	Auditory Discrimination
Auditory Figure-Ground	Auditory Identification
Auditory Localization	Auditory Memory (short term)
Auditory Memory (long term)	Auditory Monitoring
Auditory Reception	Auditory Segmentation
Auditory Sequencing	Auditory Synthesis
Auditory Vigilance	

attach the wrong sounds or meanings to the printed symbol. This child may be insensitive to rhymes and therefore will be unable to pick out words that rhyme or supply words to rhyme. Sound-blending skills, which require a child to listen to the pronunciation of a word sound-by-sound and blend the sounds mentally into a meaningful unit, may also be impaired.

Auditory Association

Auditory association occurs when attention and discrimination ability are intact. Auditory association is necessary if a child is to use received sound for language purposes. Associating sound with meaning is the key to language growth and academic success. When a child cannot associate a sound sequence with a particular experience or referent, such as a picture, word, or feeling, difficulty recalling and sequencing events occurs. When a meaning cannot be associated with a particular sound, confusion is created and a child may respond inappropriately.

The child with an auditory association problem may have difficulty in responding readily, completing sentences, or remembering simple words. He or she may require a long time to "think" of the appropriate word. This same child will fail to recognize absurdities and will not understand subtle humor. Weak abstract reasoning abilities and poor concept formation may also be present. An inability to draw relationships from what is heard, to process them internally, and to respond verbally is not uncommon. This child will also have trouble in understanding relationships and making generalizations.

Auditory Memory

A deficit in auditory memory can affect both long-term retention of experiences and information and short term recall. When a child has difficulty remembering what was taught to him he cannot associate new learning to previous information. Inability to store and retrieve auditory information effects the child's sequencing skills, and synthetic ability.

Meaning is critical in regard to auditory memory. Material that is more meaningful to the child is retained better when working with a child with auditory memory deficits. He or she may not remember names of people or objects—even those that should be familiar. Rote sequences, including the alphabet, multiplication tables, addresses, phone numbers, etc., may be difficult to learn and remember. This child may also have word-finding difficulties and be unable to supply the word to unfamiliar poems or stories that would generate meaning. In other words, these children cannot guess at unfamiliar words from the context. There may be more problems with nonmeaningful units and long term rather than short-term memory tasks.

Auditory Figure-Ground

When a child can attend, discriminate, and is able to relate sound experience to meaning but has extreme difficulty doing any of these functions in the presence of a competing background noise, an auditory figure-ground disorder is suspected. This child is unable to block out irrelevant auditory information that impacts on learning. She/he is distracted by background noise, and is unable to follow the teacher's instructions in a classroom situation. Children with auditory figure ground problems do best in quiet listening environments and on a one-to-one basis.

This child may ask for repetition when oral directions are given at home and in the classroom. His or her responses can also be totally unrelated to the original question or topic of conversation. Television may be much more enjoyable than radio or listening to a story read aloud. This youngster may repeat what is heard but cannot really understand it. Gestures may be used to replace words and to convey meaning. Multiple-meaning words will be difficult to define. These deficits lead to problems expressing emotions.

Auditory Synthesis

Auditory synthesis or closure is related to the ability to fill in the missing parts. Recognizing words, sounds, etc., when they are presented in an unorganized, incomplete, or distorted manner amid distracting or confusing noise is an example of auditory synthesis. Auditory closure is necessary in sound-blending skills and is therefore important to spelling, reading, and writing. A child with poor closure skills can have word-order problems or omit words when repeating sentences. Unfamiliar speech is difficult for this child to understand. Difficulties in understanding the relationship between concepts leads to a poor grasp of cause and effect relationships. Difficulties in sequencing events may also be noted.

Auditory synthesis is closely related to reading and spelling skills. The child may have difficulty recognizing the same sounds in different words, may have trouble dividing words into syllables, may misspell or omit words; and may be unable to blend familiar sounds to produce a correct production. Word-attack skills are usually poor. Deficits in the area lead to difficulties in perceiving parts as they relate to the whole.

Attention Deficit Disorder with and without Hyperactivity

A specific auditory disorder encompassing a number of deficient auditory processes previously described is currently known/labeled as Attention Deficit Disorder with or without Hyperactivity. Attention Deficit Disorder (ADHD) has enjoyed such popularity that it has been incorporated into the *Diagnostic and Statistical Manual III-R* (1987)[19] *[DSM-III-R]* of the American

Psychiatric Association as a diagnostic entity in its own right. It is defined as: "developmentally inappropriate degrees of inattention, impulsiveness, and hyperactivity" (p. 50). The authors have chosen to discuss this specific disorder not only because of its popularity but also because the behaviors are addressed without consideration of the underlying disordered processes. The manual suggests that there are other complicating features that vary with age such as low self-esteem, low frustration tolerance, mood lability, and temper outbursts. The disorder is seen as common and present in as much as 3 percent of school-age children in the United States. While this is but a rough estimate of incidence from research studies whose percentages range from 1–10, in England the estimate of ADHD is 0.1 percent.[20]

> In England the schools seem to do less initiating and when they do, the referral is more likely to a school psychologist or a Child Guidance Clinic. There seems to be less "medicalizing" of the problem than is usual in the United States. Another factor may be the use of DSM-III-R vs ICD-9 (International Classification of Diseases—9th Revision). Someone suggested that DSM-III is more a description of symptoms, and lists many symptoms for ADHD resulting in an increase in the number of diagnoses of ADHD. ICD-9 has tighter categories and tends to result in multiple diagnoses, so that ADHD may be a secondary diagnosis. The English school system is another factor to consider. There is more structure in the schools (as well as less violence) and fewer children are diverted out of regular classes. (p. 7)

The most consistent research finding in the incidence of ADHD is greatest in boys. A major complication of ADHD is social impairment and academic failure. The *DSM-III-R*[19] lists fourteen behavioral criteria for the diagnosis of ADHD that are presented below:

A. A disturbance of at least six months during which at least eight of the following are present:

1. Often fidgets with hands or feet or squirms in seat (in adolescents, may be limited to subjective feelings of restlessness).
2. Has difficulty remaining seated when required to do so.

3. Is easily distracted by extraneous stimuli.
4. Has difficulty awaiting turn in games or group situations.
5. Often blurts out answers to questions before they have been completed.
6. Has difficulty following through on instructions from others (not due to oppositional behavior or failure of comprehension) e.g. fails to finish chores.
7. Has difficulty sustaining attention in tasks or play activities.
8. Often shifts from one uncompleted activity to another.
9. Has difficulty playing quietly.
10. Often talks excessively.
11. Often interrupts or intrudes on others, e.g. butts into other children's games.
12. Often does not seem to listen to what is being said to him or her.
13. Often loses things necessary for tasks or activities at school or at home (e.g. toys, pencils, books, assignments).
14. Often engages in physically dangerous activities without considering possible consequences (not for the purpose of thrill seeking) e.g. runs into the street without looking.

B. Onset before the age of seven.
C. Does not meet the criteria for a Pervasive Developmental Disorder (pp. 52-52).

Although a preponderance of psychologists and psychiatrists would affirm the existence of ADHD, reviews of research and other writings on this topic suggest that whether such a distinctive disorder exists is open to question as the major symptoms of impulsivity, restlessness, and inattention are found in many other disorders of childhood. In addition, the fourteen criteria for the diagnosis of ADHD listed above are committee and politically determined and hence are arbitrarily included; they are the overt symptoms of the problem and not the problem itself. As Kohn[21] has stated:

> Those in the field accept as common knowledge that symptoms of hyperactivity often vanish when a child is watching TV, engaged in free play or doing something else he likes. Similarly, the way a child's environment is organized and the way tasks are presented

> can mean the difference between normal behavior and behavior called hyperactive, a finding that has been replicated again and again. This is particularly true for the symptoms related to paying attention. (p. 93)

Hyperactivity can therefore be said to occur when the child does not conform to the classroom (teacher) expectations.

ADHD seems to be a behavioral reaction to a very high level of anxiety whether in a child or an adult. The anxiety, especially in children, seems to be related to a number of parameters. Among them are:

1. The child's inability to understand the requirements of social interactions.
2. The inability to behave in an effective and competent manner.
3. The inability to get positive reactions from the important adults in the environment.
4. The inability to understand what is figure and what is ground in the auditory environment.
5. The inability to understand directions.
6. The inability to retain information.

This is only a partial listing. However, any one of these symptoms can raise a child's anxiety level to unbearable heights. At the anxiety levels these children function, behavioral and cognitive disruptions are inevitable. These children cannot sit still, have poor concepts of cause-effect relationships, cannot follow through on tasks, get lost in their fantasies, are very distractible, etc. Again the list can go on and on. It is not surprising that when these children are in a quiet place, or in a one-on-one situation, all the behaviors so typically described as part of the ADHD syndrome are quiescent. In these situations the child's abilities to attend and follow are not being stressed, there is the possibility of succeeding and of maintaining interpersonal connections plus a considerable reduction in the possibility of being judged as a failure and rejected. It is the failure and the rejection that these children consistently experience that can raise the anxiety level to such perilous proportions. The threat of abandonment by parents, other adults, and peers for behaviors considered, by these important people, to be unacceptable is so devastating to these children that problematic skills are further eroded.

Ritalin and Cylert are two drugs often used to reduce the symptoms of hyperactivity. However, research findings indicate that children are not slowed down so much as the behaviors are redirected. Activity may be more goal oriented and attention better sustained. The aggressivity often expressed by these children may also be reduced, peer relationships may improve, and the teacher may be able to handle the youngster more effectively. Nevertheless, assessment of research[21] during the decades of the 70s and 80s indicate that for 25–40 percent of the children medication has no effect, and of the remaining 60–75 percent a large proportion improve on a placebo, and some get worse. The research also indicates that while children may get better grades on the drugs, academic achievement is not enhanced. This is a placebo effect underscoring the fact that medication does not remedy cognitive defects nor increase the development of skills. Medication may help reduce high anxiety levels but it is by no means a cure. Rather, the underlying issues of emotional problems, language, and CAP difficulties seen in children diagnosed as ADHD need to be addressed. The development of skills to deal with the world rather than the masking of symptoms provides the child with strategies to handle learning and social interactions and leads to success.

Summary

The auditory component is especially important in the classroom in the areas of reading and language comprehension. The child in the school setting with auditory deficits will have trouble responding appropriately to auditory stimuli, organizing items correctly, and understanding the meaning of them. Auditory learning cannot be separated from other aspects of development. Auditory responses are an integral part of visual perception, emotional status, and intellectual growth. The child with auditory problems cannot discriminate and or associate sounds with selected objects or experiences. He or she may react by ignoring the auditory message or overresponding to sounds and demonstrating hyperactive behavior.[18] The way in which a youngster receives and organizes and utilizes auditory stimulation has a direct relationship to his or her future level of language learning and academic achievement.

The identification of a central auditory problem is a most complicated one that defies measurement with traditional tools. A thorough understanding of speech and language development and its relationship to auditory processing is critical in order to identify these learning problems and formulate therapeutic techniques. Chapter 2 will explore normal speech and language development and chapter 3 will discuss emotional and cognitive development.

2

Speech and Language Development

The way a family uses *language* will determine the *communication* styles of the next generation. It is also a way in which one generation transmits its culture to another.[1]

It is important to understand that there is a difference between *speech* and language. Language is a system that is represented by a number of *symbols* and is not necessarily verbal. Language may include hand signs and nonverbal body language such as facial expressions and body stance. Verbal language is also represented by words that are mutually understood by both the speaker and the listener. It is necessary for the people who are communicating with one another to understand what the verbal symbols represent.

Speech on the other hand is composed of a number of isolated sounds or *phonemes*. In the English language, there are approximately forty-five different sounds. The sounds of a language are not the same as the alphabet. There are twenty-six letters in the alphabet. The letters do not necessarily stand for or represent particular sounds.

Language makes speech possible, even though we can have language without speech. Language develops internally and may even begin before birth. In the preceding chapter on Auditory Development it was noted that children's hearing is totally intact some months before they are born and which may allow infants to recognize many elements of speech at birth.

Development of Language and Coordination

The development of communication appears to follow a regular schedule with acquisition occurring in a fairly orderly process paralleling the development of motor abilities.[2,3,4] In the first two years of life, a child is transformed from a helpless infant into a mobile communicative youngster who is intent upon exploring his/her social and physical surroundings. The two most dramatic occurrences during this early development are the onset of walking and the emergence of speech. Even though each child develops language in her/his own unique way, there are regularities in language development that are linked to motor growth.[5]

At about six months when the child begins to sit alone, an increase in babbling called *prespeech* occurs. (E.g., Mariah at six-and-one-half months can sit up and grab an object to put in her mouth. Her babbling appears to be used to get attention and express her wants. She is aware of other's speech and seems to babble in a social context.) At a year when the infant stands and begins to walk, meaningful words are also produced. By the time the infant is eighteen months, he or she is walking alone and is generally uttering one- and two-word phrases (e.g., "Dada, Mama," "Aga (all gone)," "Meer (come here)." Some children may acquire a number of words all at once and then may not show a rapid growth for some time while others slowly add words to their vocabulary. When there is significant delay in motor development, such as when the child is slow in sitting, slow in crawling, and slow in walking, there may also be an associated delay in the development of speech.[6] For example:

> Caroline at ten months was walking alone. By the time she was twelve months old she had a vocabulary of twelve words. Most of her words were associated with movements and gestures, i.e., "No" was accompanied by head movement while "Hi" and "Bye" had hand gestures along with the correct vocalization. When asked, "What does Daddy say?" Caroline shook her head and also pointed her finger while saying "No, no, no!" She was also able to execute appropriate movements in response to her mother's recitation of "Little Miss Muffett" (sitting, eating, running, etc.).

Table 2 describes language and motor development intercoordination.

TABLE 2

Simultaneous Development of Language and Coordination.
(Adapted from Emerick and VanRiper[7])

Age in Months	*Vocalization and Language*	*Motor Development*
4	Cooing sounds.	Head self-supported; sits with pillow props on three sides.
6 to 9	Babbling begins; produces sounds such as "ma" or "da"; or "ma ma," "da da."	Sits alone; pulls to standing position; first finger-thumb opposition of grasp appears.
12 to 18	Pronounces a few "words"; follows simple commands and responds to "no."	Stands alone; creeps; takes a few steps when hands are held; grasp, and release fully developed.
18 to 21	At 18 months has about 20 words in vocabulary which expands to over 200 by 21 months; points to objects; understands simple questions; uses two-word phrases.	Walks stiffly; sits on a small chair with only "fair aim," creeps downstairs backward; has trouble building a tower of three cubes; can awkwardly throw a ball.
24 to 27	Child has a vocabulary of nearly 400 words; has two- to three word phrases; uses prepositions and pronouns.	Runs but falls easily turning; can suddenly alternate between standing, kneeling and sitting positions; walks up and downstairs, one foot forward.
30 to 33	Increase in vocabulary; three- to four-word sentences; most utterances are unlike	Hand-finger coordination; manipulation of objects

TABLE 2 *(continued)*

Age in Months	*Vocalization and Language*	*Motor Development*
	adult language; unique to child.	improved; builds tower of six cubes.
36 to 39	Vocabulary of more than 1000 words; complex grammatical rules are used; mistakes are less frequent; speech about 90 percent understandable.	Walks stairs by alternating feet; jumps on one foot; can ride tricycle; can stand on one foot for a few seconds.

There has been controversy as to how much early babbling (the early sounds of the infant) actually contributes to speech and language development. In recent years it is thought that this is important to speech development. The interest in babbling is not so much in the sounds the child makes but that children all over the world sound the same during their first three months of life. If you were to listen to a child in Japan or Africa, there would be very little difference in the sounds that the children from these two areas make, similarly they would not sound different from infants of the same age in the United States.[2]

At around four or five months the child begins to make sounds representative of the sounds that he or she hears within his/her environment. In this prelanguage stage, we hear what are called comfort sounds and cooing sounds. Many of the early ones are *reflexive*. As infants grow, they practice babbling with a consonant and vowel sound. Some intonation patterns are evident as you hear a rising and falling in vocalizations. The child appears to be talking and parents respond as if the babbling were meaningful and communicative.[8] Some parents can distinguish if their baby is hungry or in pain, on the basis of the sounds he/she is making. Psychologists have stated that infants, even less than one day old, can distinguish their own cry from that of other babies. When they hear themselves on tape, they immediately quiet. Studies done with mother's voices have led researchers to conclude infants can recognize their mother's voice to the exclusion of all others. This phenomenon would support the premise that they do indeed hear before birth.[9]

> Kathryn, a three-day-old infant, is crying in her cradle. When her mother comes near and talks to her in a soft, soothing voice, Kathryn immediately stops crying.

Infants at three or four months spend time in vocal play when they are alone. This behavior often disappears when someone comes in or attracts their attention. Deaf babies also babble, but since they cannot hear the sounds they produce, they lose interest in this activity by about eight months and become silent.

In order to understand acquisition of speech and language, it is necessary to discuss it in orderly segments. However, one step does not begin and another one cease. The activity of one stage leads into the characteristics of another and the patterns of both stages can exist simultaneously. The child must hear, must practice, and must experiment in order to develop his or her own language system.

> Thirteen-month-old Margaret had a special attraction to her grandfather. During a holiday visit Margaret's grandfather made repeated attempts to teach her to say the difficult-to-pronounce word "grandpa." Just before her bedtime, Margaret looked at her grandfather and to his delight, said "Papa." The next morning, Margaret's parents reported that they heard her repeating "Papa," "Papa" over and over again as she was alone in her crib. Later that same day, she received another visit from her grandfather. She immediately extended her arms to him and said, "Papa." Of course she received immediate reinforcement from her ecstatic grandfather.

This scenario is a good example of the steps in mastering a meaningful word, i.e., producing the sounds to the word *papa,* storing sounds in memory, associating with something or someone (grandfather), and then being able to retrieve and use in a meaningful way ("Papa"). In addition, a child will learn to associate the visual expression on the parent's face with the sounds, intonations and gestures the parent is using.

Sound Development

Vowels are the first sounds the infant makes. Vowels produced in the back of the mouth are said first, such as the *oo* in sh*oe*. The first consonants on the other hand are lip sounds, such as, the *m* in mama, *b* in bye-bye, *p* in papa. Certain sounds appear before others in the child's early words. Repetitive sequences begin to emerge during the end of the first year when sounds may be said again and again, i.e., mama, dada, bye-bye. This leads to the development of a rhyme or contrasting sound by the end of the first year. It is felt that the child appears to be practicing little units of language in preparation for putting them into words and eventually sentences.[10]

Earlier in this chapter, the sound system was defined as a series of phonemes. Phonemes can be described as the building blocks for the communication of ideas.[11] From a larger repertoire of possible sounds, children learn to communicate with a basic set of sounds or phonemes appropriate to their language that are learned during the first few years of life. Sound development continues through the age of six years, but the majority of sounds are mastered by age four. In Table 3 below is a listing of phonemes and the ages at which they are mastered.

Before children freely master the sounds of language, they often substitute an early-produced sound for one that is difficult to produce, for example:

"Yook at da twain doe too too."
(Look at the train go choo choo.)
"Peaze tay home wib me."
(Please stay home with me.)

Most children's errors in speech are developmental. This means that they will probably "outgrow" them by the time they complete the second grade. However, not all speech/language difficulties will be outgrown.

First Words

The first vowel or consonant vowel combinations are produced early. The child is likely to repeat or whisper combinations like

TABLE 3

Children's mastery of phonemes, according to age
(Adapted from Meynuk,[12] 1971)

Age of Mastery	*Phonemes*
3 years	/b/,/m/,/n/,/f/,/w/,/h/
4 years	/p/,/d/,/g/,/k/,/y/(yellow),/l/,/t/
5 years	/v/,/s/,/z/,/r/
6 years	/j/(junk)
6+ years	thumb this sing

"pa" or "da" or "dada" or "baba." Oftentimes parents are asked, "When did your child say his or her first words?" The usual response is six months. However, the meaningful use of words does not begin until a year to fifteen months of age.[13] Before this time, children are practicing sounds only. At about a year the baby uses words to label or name objects in a truly meaningful manner. Words are understood long before they are actually produced. The child shows this understanding by his/her behavior. As a way of enhancing the understanding of the baby, parents tend to speak to their children in single words and short phrases, otherwise labeled as nursery language or motherese.[14] That adults reduce their speech to the level at which a child can understand is a naturally occurring phenomenon that is also seen in an older child talking to a younger one.

The first words that children use are called sentence words. The baby says "Bye-bye?" with an upward intonation of the voice and then looks toward the door or may pick up his or her jacket and crawl over to the stroller and say, "Bye-bye." The meaning conveyed is "Is it time to go?" or "Can I go?" These simple words are stated as whole sentences or whole thoughts and interpreted as such by the caretaker. They emerge very early in the pattern of language development and they will continue until the child begins to put two words together.

At about eighteen months children begin to join words together. This accomplishment is an important developmental milestone.[15,16] These two-word utterances mark the beginning of the development of *syntax*, i.e., children begin to order words in a meaningful way. At this same time, the child can begin to follow directions, perhaps two-step directions, "Go in the bedroom and get your ball." Children also appear to be able to differentiate words that refer to things, words that are labels, and words that need a *modifier.* One of the earliest modifier words is *more* which children learn can be attached to words such as *milk, candy, ball, bye-bye,* etc. The content of first words are usually things, persons, actions, and events closely related to the child's immediate life.

Development of Syntax

As stated above, at approximately eighteen months of age, children begin to join words together to form two-word utterances.[7] The following description demonstrates development of syntax.

> During the first few months of his second year, Joseph produced only single word utterances. "Bye-bye" was a command as well as a question. He sometimes said "no," "mama" or "daddy" and had approximately twenty-five words at eighteen months, including *cat, dog, baby, shoe, open, more, eat, cookie, go, down, up, on, off.* By twenty months he was combining words into unique utterances like: "more on," "bye-bye car," "more dog." Joseph also demonstrated that he learned how words could be used: "bebe (baby) eat," "dit (sit) dare (chair)" within a six-month period. Joseph remained at this level while his vocabulary acquisition increased. He expanded into three word utterances, "mama dribe (drive) tar (car)," "coat go bye," "go daddy trut (truck)."

The rate of acquisition of words can vary as do the words themselves but nonetheless there is a pattern. Brown[15] discovered that as a child's length of utterance or sentence increases, his or her language increases in complexity. By the time a child is ready to enter kindergarten, he or she will have acquired almost the entire repertoire of adult grammar. Table 4 shows the pattern in which young children acquire syntax.

Development of Semantics (Meaning)

One of the least understood aspects of children's development is how meanings are attached to the structures (syntax) of language. People associate word meaning with a dictionary type of definition. However, as words develop meaning for a youngster, he or she must have a concept of the permanence of recurring objects. The child must understand that the moon seen in the sky tonight is the same moon that was there last night and that there are not two moons or sixty moons.[11,16] A child must realize that the sandwich eaten for lunch is not the same sandwich eaten for lunch yesterday but another sandwich. The child's word for "Mama" is not a label for his or her mother until he or she learns the difference between "my mama," "not my mama," etc. When a child understands what the various uses of a

TABLE 4

Acquisition of Syntax
(Adapted from Brown, 1973)[15]

1. Present progressive—"ing" ending on verb. Children use this first without auxiliary (helping) verb: "Me sitting," "Me eating," "Her crying."

2–3. In, on—these are prepositions used frequently by most children in early speech. "Baby on chair," "Cat in bed."

4. Plural—(regular and irregular forms) "cookies," "men."
5. Past irregular—includes "got," "went," "came," "fell," "broke," "sat."
6. Possessive—"mama's," "kitty's."
7. "To be" verb used to connect subject and object. "What is this?" or "I be bad," "Me be good."
8. "A," "the," appearing before common nouns: "a lot," "the baby."
9. Past regular—"d" endings on verbs: "pulled," "washed."
10. S endings on third-person verbs: "pulls," "washes."
11. Third-person irregular forms—"is," "has," "does."
12. Auxiliary verbs—for example, she is running home.
13. Contractible copula—contracted forms of #7: "What's this?" or "It's mine."
14. Contractible auxiliary verbs—for example: "She's running home."

word imply, the child has developed a concept to go with a particular label. A child must also develop a connection between a label and a thing-that is, between the word *cookie* and the actual object. A working concept must be in place before a child can appropriately classify all the objects in his or her world.[16]

> Caroline associated the word "car" only with her father's truck. Soon she applied the word to all cars and trucks and vans. She then used "car" to label everything with wheels that moved. Caroline was then able to distinguish trucks from cars and then was able to separate van as another category. Caroline needed to understand that all moving things with wheels are not necessarily cars and could not be identified by a single one word or one attribute.

Children appear to develop semantic concepts through experience with the environment as well as through trial and error. When children first begin to talk, they express what they know from their own experiences.[17] They must then be able to organize these experiences in such a way that they can communicate this knowledge to others through language.

> Fifteen-month-old David was sitting high on his father's shoulders during a walk across the neighborhood late one afternoon. He was interested in everything as demonstrated by his constant chatter. As they walked along, David looked up at a tall tree, pointed his arm upward and said: "Tree very up there."

This is an example of how early concepts develop when the child's language is not complex enough to explain these concepts. The child produces unique utterances that have been constructed out of the child's own experience with a particular concept.

> Three-year-old Richard lived in an older home in a neighborhood with a number of retired couples. He was befriended by an older man, Mr. Smith, who lived around the corner. One day in a conversation with his mother Richard described the retiree as "you know Mr. Smith everyday is his day off!"

In these examples, David's concept of high and Richard's concept of retired were expressed in terms that matched their own unique experiences and their language development.

Reception of sensory input from hearing, seeing, feeling and tasting along with active experiences with the environment provide the basis for early categorization and organization.[18,19]

> Joseph at twenty months was sitting in his high chair eating supper when he heard an airplane fly over his house. He stopped eating, pointed upward and said, "Airplane." His mother who was feeding him, responded; "yes, that is an airplane." Joseph continued pointing upward and then said, "Moon?" (using a rising intonation to reflect a question). Joseph was associating the airplane in the sky with his experience of also seeing the moon in the same sky. He, at this young age, is appropriately classifying objects in his world.

The young child does not passively wait to hear and learn words or anything else. He or she is an active developing interactive human being. The meaning of language for the child arises from interactions with the environment and is a continuation of development that began in early infancy. Table 5 represents examples of early semantic development.

Development of Pragmatics

Pragmatics is concerned with how language is used to communicate in interpersonal situations. In every kind of daily situation there are dynamics that affect us. If we step into an elevator we usually do not talk, we are usually silent and we stare at the indicator that tells us what floor we are on. When we meet somebody for the first time, we usually talk about general things, for example, the weather, our children, or current events. We are all aware of the rules of social interaction, which we have been learning since the day we were born. That we typically and consistently follow these rules without even being aware of them demonstrates that they are used implicitly.[11]

Learning pragmatics is a lifelong task. However, children indicate an awareness of it at a very early age. Even small children speak differently to strangers than to their parents. They speak differently to an infant, to a baby-sitter, to their stuffed animal, or to an imaginary playmate. They also speak differently to the same people in different situations. For example, the way chil-

TABLE 5

Development of Meaning
(Adapted from Wood, 1976[11])

Preword Stage	Intonations that are accompanied by gestures.
Nonstandard Word Stage	"Baby talk," Infant refers to a particular item which is accompanied by an appropriate intonation.
Single-Word Stage (i.e., "cookie")	Child produces understandable words.
Two-Word Stage	Child says "daddy cookie" pointing and intonation patterns remain. Child knows what she/he wants.
Object-Action Stage	Child begins conversation "drink milk," "eat cookie," "doggy go nite nite," child comments about objects, people, and events.
Mature Stage	Child uses question intonation, pattern (use at end of sentence) good manners to perform intentional social behaviors.

dren speak to their mothers during meal time is much different from the way they speak when they are having a bath or going for a walk. Children have learned to adjust their speech and behavior to various situations even though they are still learning the rules and the sounds of their language.

> Eighteen-month-old Joseph was visiting his grandparents. He spotted his grandfather's open briefcase stuffed with papers. Joseph apprehensively reached for the briefcase with an eye on his grandfather, and seemed to be waiting for a sign of his approval or disapproval. Joseph's mother was observing the scene and remarked that if the child were in his own home and the briefcase belonged to Daddy, Joseph would have it emptied in seconds! Joseph is demonstrating the way in which even very young children adjust their behavior to different situations.

There are five functions of communication for pragmatics and are usually expressed in everyday communication.[20,21,22,10] They are as follows:

1. Informing
2. Controlling or persuading
3. Expressing one's feelings
4. Performing communicative rituals
5. Performing imaginary events/play.

Informing

The information function probably is the easiest of all functions to talk about. Everyone seems to understand that people interact and exchange information. It is assumed that information is an early function to emerge in children, however it does emerge quite late. Haliday[23] notes that some informative utterances are the last to appear. In order to get information to someone else, you must tell them something that you know that they do not. It emerges late because the child has to understand something about differences between him-herself and others. They must also understand how to communicate knowledge, and within this context, the give and take of a conversation.

Controlling

Persuading, arguing, convincing, nagging, and/or begging, are control kinds of strategies. A parent who punishes a child for using bad language is exercising control.

Expressive Feelings

A child might tell her friend "I'm mad that you won't give me one." There is information in this statement, but there is also some controlling, as well as expression of feelings.

Communication Rituals

This involves all ceremonies such as religious rites, pledging allegiance, prayers before meals and after meals. Greetings such as "How are you today?" "I am fine" are also ritualized. Ritualistic communications are in games that mothers and children play, such as peekaboo, I'm hiding this, where did I put it? and patty-cake. These are ritualistic games and they appear to train the child to anticipate new information as he or she develops language.[21]

Imagining

Imagining is somewhat different from all the other functions. The function of imagination tells the child that this is not real, it is make-believe and would fall under pretending. Children generally do well at this and included in this are story telling, acting, making believe, and other forms of play.

Play

People are slow to recognize the importance of the imagining function in children's development. Pretending and playing is an excellent indication that they are developing representations of ideas about reality. At the later ages they engage in rehearsal, sometimes dress rehearsal of things they want to say or roles they want to play. This process is learned extremely early. Researchers feel that imagining and role playing relate to learning about the future and about abstract kinds of concepts.[11] Children must be encouraged to play, imagine, and be creative since these skills will manifest themselves later in life and are the underpinnings for critical thinking tasks, problem solving, and abstractions. Engaging in play allows children to make decisions about what the world is really like.

Through play children learn that language is not only a tool for communication, but also for learning that facilitates higher levels of thinking as the child grows older.

Pragmatics develop from the earliest infant caretaker interactions to a higher level of mastery in adulthood. For some, pragmatic development continues throughout their entire life span. Early pragmatic development appears to occur as a result of direct environmental feedback.[24] For example,

> During a birthday party for his great aunt, two and a half year old Patrick says, "Me want cake." His mother who does not allow him to eat sweets ignores her son. Patrick pulls on his mother's arm and gives her this verbal plea, "Me want cake please." Patrick's

mother replies, "Cake is not healthy for little boys." Patrick persists and changes his tone and says "Me want cake please thank you."

The result of including all the appropriate social rules earned Patrick a small piece of the prized birthday cake. Patrick was able to comply with what he knew his mother expected in social rules and as a result was able to achieve his desire for a rare treat.

Pragmatics develops very rapidly in the intermediate years when the child goes to school. School is a very important setting for learning cultural and social messages. During the intermediate years pragmatic problems may become apparent. This may lead to arrests in later development. Problems with pragmatics cause significant peer relationship difficulties. Sometimes the pragmatic problems are difficult to identify because the behaviors may be seen as unrelated to language. For example, a child may be accused of being rude because he/she says to the teacher: "I don't want to do my school work." The child may not understand what is required of him/her but the teacher gets angry at the way in which he/she has spoken and may say, "Don't sass me!" The child has not identified the rules and certainly does not understand how things went wrong. He/she may be punished by the teacher, the principal, and perhaps even the parents without really understanding why. This type of distinctive interaction will be discussed further in subsequent chapters.

Adequate pragmatic abilities enable children to become effective communicators. Without these abilities children fail in communication at all levels. Failure in pragmatics can also be the foundation for more severe problems. For example, lack of pragmatic ability can contribute to failures in areas other than academic achievement because it interferes with the gains of positive reactions from social interactions. Deviant pragmatic development can result in children becoming unable to fit into the social environment and may also contribute to low self esteem.[25] The child with pragmatic difficulty may be perceived by others as incapable of taking part in desired or appropriate social interaction. The self-fulfilling negative image can in many ways perpetuate pragmatic deficits. Appropriate learning cannot be achieved when a child has inadequate pragmatic development that leads to failures in understanding subtle messages conveyed by teachers in the classroom or by peers.[26]

School-Age and Adult Speech and Language Development

Most researchers, prior to 1970, made the assumption that a child's speech and language development was completed by the time he or she entered school.[27] It is now recognized that language development continues into adulthood but the school years are much more important than originally conceptualized. As was stated earlier in this chapter, the preschool years are the critical period for language learning, however, growth continues to occur in all aspects of language; syntax, semantics, phonology, and pragmatics during the school years. The child adds new structures and refines and expands existing forms. These developments assist the child to express more complex relationships and to use language in much more creative and complex ways.

During the school-age period as well as the adult years, the individual increases the size of his or her vocabulary that includes the understanding of specific word definitions. Abstract knowledge is increased. Individual interpretation of language and spoken and written messages also increase in the way words are used. According to Francis,[28] one major manifestation is the increase of the creative or figurative use of language to gain effect or for affect.

The period of most rapid change appears to occur between five and nine years of age when children move from preconceptual thinking to concrete operations (this will be explained fully in chapter 3). It is not until the adult years that many new associations become consistent and fully integrated. Anglin[29] states that words from a sensory domain such as "hot" and "cold" may be associated with psychological states. These associations probably are related to more figurative uses of language.

Figurative language allows the school-age child to use words in an imaginative sense rather than a literal one in order to demonstrate an emotional impression. Figurative language includes idioms, metaphors, and proverbs. For example, "hit the road," "take a hike," "bite your lip," "jump the gun." These powerful terms are not learned as part of a rule system but as a result of experience. They cannot be interpreted literally. They are acquired through continual use and their meanings are inferred from a contextual standpoint. As age increases, an individual sharpens word definitions and relationships that result in more accurate communication. Individuals also learn to use language figuratively. As a result of both processes, communication in the adult becomes more precise, flexible, and creative.

During the school years, however, the child completes phonetic development. By age eight, the child as was stated earlier in this chapter can produce all English sounds accurately.[30] This allows for development of cognitive processing, storage, and retrieval. In addition, it frees up the child to use more abstract concepts and thoughts, which in turn allows for the development of figurative language. During the school years there seems to be some change in cognitive processing storage and retrieval. This would correspond to Piaget's[31] concrete operational period, a period in which the child begins to use abstract thought. This is also discussed more completely in chapter 3.

The area of most important growth in language during the school and adult years is in use of language and pragmatic skills. During the school years, children gain the ability to clarify messages and to produce subtleties in their language. To produce clear messages the child must monitor as well as evaluate setting and cues regarding the success or failure of the communicative message. According to White,[32] the school-age child should have the following pragmatic abilities:

1. Gain and hold attention in an acceptable manner with an adult
2. Ask for information or help from others
3. Express his or her anger or affection in an appropriate manner
4. Follow peers as well as direct them
5. Tell stories in competitive situations with peers
6. Express pride in his or her accomplishments
7. Role-play.

Language is also used effectively by high school students in creative situations, in sarcasm, in jokes and also double-meaning words.[33] These skills begin to develop in the early school years. Children with language-learning disabilities often have problems in this area. As a result, peer relationships suffer or cannot be effectively developed because the language-learning disabled child is not able to interpret and understand the language environment of his or her peers.

Gender Differences

Gender differences have been recognized as early as in the middle years of elementary school. Gender differences appear to occur in vocabulary use as well as conversational style. For example, women tend to avoid coarse language in their conversations and tend to use more polite words while men tend to use more expletives.[34] Men and women also differ in both talking and turn-taking behaviors. Men tend to be more verbose than women.[35] Women's conversations with men or other women appear to be shorter. Within conversations men and women use different turn-taking styles. Adult males interrupt female speakers more often than they interrupt males and more often than females interrupt speakers of either sex. The actual basis for gender differences is actually unknown.[36]

Summary

Speech and language development is a complex process that involves motor coordination, linguistic processing, and cognitive maturation. The process begins before birth and continues throughout a lifetime. At birth speech mechanisms are used primarily for breathing and eating. The infant's crying begins to be differentiated and interpreted by the caregiver. The role of hearing becomes important in the development of early sound production. The child begins to understand words and gestures that are accompanied by progressive motor development. Receptive language acquisition continues as the child begins to produce single words. Vocabulary expands rapidly, speech becomes more understandable as the child eventually speaks in sentences of six or more words. By age five the child has acquired much of the structure of a major language user.[37] Speech and language development continues, however, as the child gains skill in pronouncing the sounds of his or her language adding new grammatical structures and has skill in transmitting communication effectively. Language development continues throughout life especially in the semantic aspects and acquisition of vocabulary.

Why Children Learn to Communicate

For years it was assumed that children acquired language because they were good learners and parents provided good reinforcements for speaking. Results of recent research in the areas of child development and speech pathology support the theory that children's language acquisition reflects the uniqueness of the human brain and its power to acquire this remarkable symbol system. Language acquisition helps prepare a child to shift from the family to wider social contacts and finally to the classroom. Language is fundamental to all academic subjects.[1]

The fact that human babies are born into a species of speaking individuals is important to the understanding of speech and language acquisition. Children acquire language because they are human. According to Piaget,[31] this is a result of the general process of cognitive development. Children learn to speak as a component of learning to think as human beings.

In the process of learning language, children share a common birthright, but each child must encounter that process as an individual. Any theory of communication development must include the processes of how children experience communication events and how they learn. Children's progress in language acquisition is a result of their unique learning strategies.[38] Looking at learning strategies is important to educators, therapists, and parents because these individuals are all concerned with why some children communicate more effectively than others.

3

Cognitive and Emotional Development of Children

Piaget, who was a professor at the University of Geneva, spent over fifty years talking to children and developing theories of *cognitive development* that have been widely accepted throughout the world. Considered a leading authority in the field of cognitive child development, he focused mainly on the development of remembering, reasoning, and believing within the context of logical thinking. While he did not pay much attention to emotional development he did suggest that the child's intellectual level enables certain types of emotional functioning. Even though a child may have had an experience with the death of a pet or a grandparent before the age of seven, a basic understanding of death is not possible because the cognitive structures necessary for understanding death have not yet been developed. For example:

> Freddy and Jan (aged four) had been playing death and dying games since Jan's grandmother had died six months previously. This day they had spread out two posters on the floor, lain down on them, and covered themselves individually with another set of posters. Jan said, "Are you dead yet, Freddy?" Freddy said, "No, are you?" Jan replied, "You can't be dead yet 'cause you're moving your foot." And the conversation went back and forth in this manner for a while before the two children shifted to another, more fruitful game.

It is quite apparent that the children had been given some information about death but they had not fully integrated the information and did not really understand death. Their cognitive level was not sufficiently developed to cope with issues of death. For Piaget, this would be an example of the child's inability to deal with emotional material that is beyond her/his ability to think, communicate, and understand. However, concentration on just cognitive growth, without consideration of emotional development, gives us only a limited picture of how children grow. Emotional development must be considered in its own right and in interaction with cognition to give a full picture of development. A discussion of cognitive development will be presented first, followed by the most prevalent theory of emotional development, that of Erik Erikson, a child analyst.

Cognitive Development

Sensorimotor Stage (birth–2 Years)

The first stage of cognitive development, the sensorimotor period, according to Piaget[1] begins at birth and lasts until the child is approximately two years of age. The cognitive development that occurs during this period is based upon the inborn reflexes of the individual (e.g., the startle reflex, the hand to mouth reflex, etc.). Connections and elaborations of these reflexes develop in the course of interaction with the environment during these early months. Since those areas of the brain necessary for long-term memory and the retrieval of memories are not developed until the end of the first year of life,[2] the memory that we see in very young children is based upon recognition. We as adults have similar experiences such as when we see someone we know we have seen before but cannot remember where or when we saw them, or even recall the name. Through a variety of experiences during the first year of life the child learns about cause-effect relationships, turn taking, self-control, and use of language while she/he is being cared for and played with by the important people in her/his environments.

By the end of the first year children are typically beginning to produce single words that have a variety of meanings. (See chapter 2.) It is during the second year of life when language is beginning that truly intelligent behavior develops. For Piaget,[1] true intelligence is expressed in experimentation. Babies experiment with their toys, with people, and other objects in the environment. For example:

> A 14-month-old had been put down for his afternoon nap, and as usual Mother would hear much movement from his room as this child typically rocked in his crib before falling asleep. He soon quieted and mother did her typical chores free from the distraction of a very exploratory toddler. When the child did not seem to awaken from his nap at his usual time Mother went to check on him but was unable to open his bedroom door fully. Through a two inch opening she had managed to effect, the mother found that the child had rocked his crib clear across the room and the bars had become wedged under the door knob. He had opened the doors to his chest and had pulled all his clothes out. A pile of clothing was in his bed, some draped over his head as though he had been attempting to try them on by himself. Mother found a broom and used it to press against the lever that held the bars in an upright position hoping to drop the side and free it from the doorknob. Mother was not able to unwedge the crib side until the youngster had concluded his experimentation with the broom handle (e.g., pushed, bitten, and played).

The intellectual development that occurs during these two years of life is dependent upon the child's acting upon the environment as described in the vignette above. This growth is also dependent upon *assimilation* and *accommodation* that create continuous changes in the intellectual structure of the person throughout his/her whole life span.

Assimilation is a process whereby the individual assumes that the new material she/he is learning can be incorporated into the information he/she already knows without it changing preconceived notions. For example:

> A five-year-old had come home from school where her kindergarten class had been talking about mommy alligators and daddy alligators making baby alligators. Her mother thought that the child was somewhat confused about her information and questioned her regarding where/how the daddy alligator carried the "seed" necessary to making a baby alligator. After careful thought the youngster very definitively told her mother that the daddy

alligator carried the seed in his back paw and walked very carefully on it so as not to hurt the seed.

Clearly, this youngster was giving an explanation of carrying based upon her understanding and experiences with carrying objects herself. Her understanding had not yet shifted to accommodate the new information. She extended her understanding to include the new information (assimilation) but had not yet altered her understanding of "carrying" (accommodation) to include other ways of carrying besides in the hand/paw. When she can broaden her concepts of carrying, as in this case to include inside the body, her conceptual system will have used accommodation in the Piagetian sense. Assimilation and accommodation are two important facets of intellectual development that we use throughout life, especially as we are learning new material.

Preconceptual Thinking (2–7 Years)

From two until about seven, according to Piaget,[1] a child's thinking is based upon visual understanding of the world and not through the careful logical thinking one comes to expect from older children and adults. Children during these ages are basically nonlogical and concrete. For example:

Three-year-old Mark had been following a leaf being blown by the wind while having a lively conversation with his father about what is alive and what is not. In response to questions he finally came to the conclusion that whatever moved was alive, what did not move was not alive but if he were sleeping and not moving he would still be alive because people are alive.

Mark was attempting to classify objects and people into the animate and inanimate even though his thinking was faulty or nonlogical and very concrete. Nevertheless, these characteristics of *preoperational* thought are necessary for continuous development, but are obstacles to logical thought. Experience and interaction with the environment enable the preconceptual child to slowly modify his/her thinking and understanding.

At this stage the *egocentricity* of the child leads her/him to the conclusion that everyone thinks in the same way and about the same thing as he or she does. During this period children do not question the validity of their thoughts because they assume that their way of understanding is the only possible way of thinking about things. For example:

> A four-year-old announced to his mother that a turtle was a big tornado because they both began with *T*. When she offered the possibility that a tornado was a big wind and the turtle an animal and that they are two separate things he disagreed with her and opined that he had thought about it and a tornado could only be a big turtle. Only time helped him to change his mind.

Piaget[1] notes that when confronted with evidence that is contradictory *preconceptual* children conclude that the evidence is wrong.

Centration is another aspect of preconceptual thinking. In centration, the child tends to fixate, or center her/his attention on a limited *perceptual* aspect of the stimulus. The child cannot decenter and thus only takes in the superficial aspects of an event. Perceptual evaluation so dominates thinking that when a series of seven pennies is placed in a line that takes up more space than a series of nine pennies placed in a line, the child will point to the longer line of seven pennies as more than the shorter line of nine pennies. This will happen even when the child knows that nine is larger than seven.

Another quality of intellectual functioning during this stage is related to the lack of reversibility in thinking. *Irreversibility* is most clearly demonstrated in the classical experiment using two different-sized glasses: after pouring the water from the tall, thin glass into the short squat glass the child is queried and will state that the tall, thin glass had more water than the short squat glass. The child cannot reverse the process to recognize that no water has been lost from the tall glass. The child cannot maintain the equivalence of amount in the face of the perceptual changes.

Concrete Operations (7–12 Years)

During these early school years, the child's thinking processes become more logical so that now when faced with a discrepancy between thought and perception, the child can draw conclusions based upon logical thinking. The major cognitive skill acquisition is reversibility. This ability involves being able to trace one's thinking from the conclusion back to the beginning, a skill that was missing during the previous stages of cognitive development. However, the child cannot yet think about unexperienced or hypothetical situations and knowledge, but rather handles concrete objects and events, directly experienced in a logical manner. Children still do not have the breadth of verbal skills necessary for in-depth explanation. In a sense then, the concrete operations child is in a transitional period between the preoperational stage and the last stage of cognitive development, formal operations.

In the concrete operation stage, the child's thinking is no longer egocentric as was found in the previous stage of development. Rather the child is aware that others can and do come to conclusions that differ from her/his own that often leads the child to look for validation of her/his thinking. Social interactions aid in the lessening of egocentric thinking and provide alternative models of thinking and knowing about the world. Concepts are developed, verified, and/or altered through social interactions. Furthermore, logical operations are no longer externalized or talked through out loud. Rather, children during this period of development can think through a problem logically and internally. Thinking has become an important skill.

Formal Operations (12 and above)

The ability to organize and play with ideas in a logical manner, especially in regard to knowledge that has not been directly experienced, becomes very important during the early phase of this stage. As most parents of a young adolescent will tell you, they are often accused of not listening by their child. The scenario usually goes something like "Mom, or Dad, if you were listening to me the only conclusion you could come to is the one I have presented to you. Therefore, if you do not agree with me you could not possibly have listened to my argument." Once again, especially with this new and last level of cognitive development there is evidence of egocentrism. Gradually, through the process of interaction with the environment the adolescent egocentrism is modified and true formal operations are acquired.

The unifying thread that runs through the cognitive development described above is the reliance upon adequate verbal language skills. While cognitive and linguistic development seem to arise from the same basic structures within the brain, after about two years they seem to take their own separate yet related courses. The interaction of language on cognition and vice versa is still not completely understood; however, cognitive and linguistic development continue to have a profound impact upon one another throughout the rest of childhood and adolescent development. Since auditory and speech/language development have been described in the two preceding chapters a discussion of the development of communication with emphasis on the cognitive emotional aspects of a child's development will be discussed.

Development of Communication

Communication is a process whereby one person shares information with another through the use of signs, symbols, words, facial, and body movement. The primary function of language according to the *Oxford English Dictionary*[3] is communication. Infants do not use words, and only slowly, and in interaction with the environment, develop consensually validated signs that convey their needs to others. Current infant research has exploded many myths about infancy and the capacity of the infant to display intentional, communicative interactions by two months. Differential behavior in interaction with mother, father, strangers, and inanimate objects has been noted. The following vignette describes communicative interaction by an infant.

> A woman I had been seeing for psychotherapy brought her three month old son to a session so that I could see the child. During the course of the session he began fussing so she breast fed him while continuing to talk with me. The child nursed for a short time and then stopped. He began cooing and looking at her very attentively. The impression I gained was of her being called by the child to pay attention to him. When this woman attended to the child he began to nurse quite contentedly. When she again talked to me, the child once again stopped nursing, calling to her. This

infant seemed to desire an interaction with his mother and could initiate a familiar pattern their usual interaction made.

Further data from infant research indicates that infants are able to modify their behaviors appropriately during social interaction. In fact, infants are capable of imitation within hours after birth.[4] This imitative skill is necessary for learning. Somewhere between eight and ten months, possibly earlier, the baby when fed with a spoon will imitate the process and feed the adult in return. When the interaction is distorted or not forthcoming, the infant often engages in behaviors that are aimed at reinstating the usual interactions.

Split-screen experiments[5] enable an examiner to watch both baby and mother simultaneously. Interactions between the two were designed to explore typical, mutual interactions. When the mother was instructed to stare straight ahead with no expression on her face the baby's reactions to this unresponsive mother were clearly noted. Researchers[5] found that the infants tried all the behaviors typical of their interactions with their mothers and when the babies could not engage their mothers, they became distressed. The organization of the baby's behavior seemed to break down (e.g., crying and fussing behaviors escalated in the baby demonstrating distress, while regression in behaviors was noted in tonguing movements, drooling, jerky hand and leg movements, and hiccuping).

Other data from split-screen experiments[5] suggest that in interaction with the primary caretaker, the baby regulates the amount of stimulation received. During play, when the baby seemed to have gotten more stimulation than she/he could manage at the time, the baby turned her/his attention away from the mother, looked at other objects or her/his own hands for a brief period and then returned her/his attention to the interaction with the mother. This type of behavior that was seen repeatedly in mother-infant dyads led researchers to the conclusion that the infant is quite capable of regulating the interpersonal interaction at a relatively early age.

The results of the experiments cited above led researchers[6] to theorize that the infant's goal is to establish mutual exchange with the primary caretaker. In fact, from birth babies scan the human face and when given a choice between a human face or an object, prefer to look at the face. By six weeks of age the baby produces an open eyed smile that typically initiates interactions with adults in the environment. Other patterns of interaction build on this, for adults talk and interact with infants as if they understand both language and facial interactions. As a result, findings from the research[7] indicate that babies, during the second six months of life, understand the rules of interpersonal play interactions. A group of ten-month-old babies played with an experimenter in a give-and-take situation for half an hour over a number of sessions. After an interval of about a week, the children were brought back to the same situation with the examiner, who did not play with them this second time. The babies initiated the same type of play they had engaged in previously. When the examiner did not respond as the babies had come to expect, they (the babies) engaged in behaviors indicating that they were taking their turn and playing for the examiner when she did not take her turn. This turn taking behavior suggested that the babies understood the rules of the interaction and could successfully enact that understanding.

Parents respond as if the birth cry was a first communication from their infant. The crying of infants alerts the interpersonal environment that there is some need that requires attention. Crying also seems to give the infant some experiential sense of mouth, tongue, lips, and palate; knowledge that may be related to the eventual development of language proper. While it takes time for mothers to become attuned to the different varieties of cries infants produce, by the time infants are four months of age, even first time mothers are consistently able to understand the meaning of the cry.[8]

Murray and Trevarthen[9] explored the impact on the interaction of mother and infant when the infant did not respond to the mother's baby talk. When the child was not responsive to the mother's interactions, they found an increase in negative comments, and mother-centered utterances (initiatives located with the mother, directives, prompt questions, calls for attention, etc.). Thus, the language of the mother became more like the language used in adult conversation. However, when the infant was responsive to the mother, there were more child-centered utterances that were related to the actions of the baby. The baby who cannot make sense of the mother's baby talk will have an even more difficult time making sense of the adultlike language the mother uses to encourage the child to respond. This may result in the baby's withdrawing attention from the interaction with mother, and others, as they are continually being overwhelmed by stimuli that they cannot handle.

Vygotsky[10,11] and Luria[12] have both suggested that from birth the mother's use of baby talk focuses the infant's attention towards objects and thus provides ways in which the infant can understand and conceptualize the world. According to Luria, language is part of development from birth. He suggested that the language of the parents, by naming and focusing the infant's attention, defines connections and relationships for the infant, shaping the processes whereby the child experiences and understands reality. He further stated that words influence the child not only by their direct impact upon perception and consciousness, but also as a regulator of behavior. Words also provide a way of ordering the world, and a means of establishing and maintaining relationships to parents and other important people in the environment. Current infant research[6] supports Luria's contention that by one to two months infants discriminate speech sounds and link sound patterns to objects. This linking of sound patterns to objects is one of the bases for the formation of adequate perception and memory. As a result of this discrimination ability infants are able to demonstrate conversationlike turn taking with their caretakers by about three months of age. Murray and Trevarthen[9] stated that there is:

> a fine sensitivity in the infant to the form, timing, and direction of adult communication, and also complex, coherently organized repertoires of expressions and behaviors that vary systematically in response to the changes in the partner's behavior. (p. 15)

Through these processes the infant learns about turn taking, the expression of needs, and responses to these expressions. Infants also begin to modify the intonations of their babbling to match those of the adult. Rising and falling patterns of intonations are discernible at about six-to-eight months, intonations typical of sentences appear at about seven months and commands at about ten months. These discriminations enable the infant and growing child to understand the subtle cues inherent in all aspects of language: content of speech, tone, gesture, and expression.

Body movement accompanies linguistic behavior in all cultures[13] and is part of the constellation of factors that are involved in learning/understanding language. Freedman[13] has suggested that bodily action has a central role in the processing of information and has been linked to measures of cognitive style and linguistic competence. This can be seen in the language-acquisition problems of the blind child and in the difficulties of the deaf child knowing what to attend to. He further suggests that the *kinesthetic* experience may be bound, along with visual images of the object, to the word(s) naming the object. This finding suggests that the communicative process, which begins in early infancy, can be disordered even before the child begins to talk as similar information is not being obtained across sense modalities.

Many theorists, Vygotsky,[10,11] Bruner,[14] Piaget,[1] to name but a few, have suggested that there is a relationship between cognitive and language development. However, to date, the nature of the relationship between cognition and language is not known. Nevertheless, Lindsay and Norman[15] in talking about the child concluded that "as his capacity to communicate symbolically develops, language and thought becomes so inextricably intermixed it becomes almost impossible to separate" (p. 437).

The ability to think symbolically begins somewhere around the second half of the second year of life, or at about eighteen months of age. *Symbolism* (a sign that stands for an object, e.g., the word *shoe* stands for the actual object) is based upon the ability to form mental representations or pictures. This ability does not usually occur before eighteen months. As previously noted, until about nine to ten months of age babies have what is called recognition memory. This form of memory enables the baby to know that it has seen or experienced something previously. Memory that enables the child to bring forth mental images does not develop until the last months of the first year of life. The learning of words to label objects in the environment, begins about a year of age and may well enhance this memory and the development of mental imagery, skills necessary for language development. The playful interactions between the infant and the primary caretaker have been crucial and relevant for the acquisition of language. The baby-mother play is usually linguistically and semantically simple, restricted, and repetitive. It usually has a well-defined structure (e.g., peekaboo, this little piggy, all around the garden), which the baby can recall as being familiar. The role structure and reciprocity is similar to the interaction or turn taking in conversation. From the beginning, the infant is flooded with language and the preparations necessary for a variety of forms of communication, but especially in the form of oral language.

At about a year children begin to use single words that name objects. Various tonal qualities in the use of the words alert caretakers as to the needs/wants of the child. By eighteen months the child has developed two word utterances that may include the noun and an adjective or a noun and a verb, and, as was mentioned above, the ability to create mental *representations* and symbolic thinking. The later-appearing abilities are enhanced with the increasing development of play, especially of symbolic play. These very important milestones develop within the context of critically important interpersonal relationships. It is here, in the early years of development that the foundations for adequate learning in school begins. White[16] suggests that by the time a child is three years of age, the interpersonal interactions she/he has experienced have already determined the kinds of grades she/he will achieve in school. He based his conclusions upon the kinds of verbal interactions the child has with her/his major caretaker. As a result we must ask ourselves how does a child become learning disabled.

The authors of this book have come to the conclusion, after working with thousands of children, that learning disabilities can begin at birth and are related to both gross and subtle difficulties in understanding language and other forms of communication. Learning disabilities are language disabilities. Children are born programmed to interact interpersonally, and to take in and process stimuli auditorially, visually, and kinesthetically. If an infant cannot process incoming stimuli interpersonal processes cannot be managed and an understanding of the world is hampered and may be distorted. Karelitz and Fisichelli[17,18] suggested that the cries and crying behavior of brain damaged infants are so variable that it would be quite difficult for mothers or caretakers to discern the problem. They found for example that normal infants respond to painful stimuli by crying more consistently, more rhythmically, and for longer periods of time than do brain damaged infants. The cries of brain-damaged children are shorter and for shorter periods of time, less rhythmic, and are more difficult to understand, not only for first time mothers, but experienced mothers as well. The inability of the mother to understand and comfort her child can and often does lead to mutual miscuing very much along the lines of the split screen experiments and the work of Murray and Trevarthen[9] described above. The difficulty in understanding the communications from important others, and the inability to understand incoming stimuli adequately interfere not only with the communicative-learning process, but also with adequate social and emotional development. How a child ideally develops will be addressed in the next section.

Emotional Development from Birth through Twelve Years of Age

According to Erikson,[19] at each stage of development there are certain critical tasks that a child must successfully master to develop in an adequate emotional manner. This mastery allows the individual to cope successfully with the next developmental crisis. The first of these tasks/stages is the development of *Trust* vs. *Mistrust*. This stage is the foundation for the remainder of emotional development. Children who exhibit language disorders at later ages have difficulty mastering the tasks of development from the beginning. They cannot trust the environment to satisfy their needs. The inability to trust the environment stems in part from the infant's difficulty in developing a sense of competence.[20] This sense of competence arises from understanding the interactions between her/himself and the caretakers in the environment. When infants understand their interactions with their caretakers they can motivate the known interaction. However, infants with language disorders often do not understand the meaning behind facial expressions and the subtle changes in oral interaction patterns; as a result they are not responsive to caretakers, who in turn gradually reduce the responsiveness to their infant. Soothing and comforting are misunderstood by both the infant and caretaker leaving the infant vulnerable and unable to develop the skills necessary for calming and soothing themselves. The environment is therefore experienced as inconsistent and nonnurturing due to the erratic experiences of these infants. Like the older language-disordered child, sometimes the information is processed, sometimes it just does not get into the system, and sometimes it is incompletely understood, all of which leads to distortions in understanding the world and the people who inhabit that world. The potentially language-disordered infant may display the varieties of communicative difficulties experienced by the older child, however, they are usually not recognized as such at this early level. As a result of environmental inconsistencies these children cannot come to rely on the environment and the important people in that environment. Basic trust cannot be fully established. The skills and achievements necessary to maneuver through the next stage, *Autonomy* vs. *Shame and Doubt,* are circumscribed and limited as the development of trust is the foundation for all other emotional development. The child, unsure of her-/himself and the important people in the world does not move out of the parent-child orbit to test her-/himself. The child cannot establish her-/himself as a separate and distinct human being with thoughts and feelings of her/his own. The struggle between closeness and separateness, which is so much a part of this stage of emotional development, cannot be resolved. On the one hand the child has not been able to master the tasks of the first stage and needs to remain at that level to finish the job, while on the other hand development pushes the child to the next stage unprepared to deal with issues of separation and separateness. The unpreparedness of these children interferes with the development of a well differentiated sense of self. Vulnerabilities in dealing with the environment develop. A sense of autonomy cannot be fostered that leads to social/interpersonal difficulties and maintains the child at an egocentric level of thinking and experiencing. As a result, the child is not prepared for the next stage of development.

During *Initiative* vs. *Guilt* the child must begin to make the appropriate sex-role identification and find her/his place both as a separate individual and as a member of an ongoing family.

Self-control, so often an issue with language-handicapped youngsters, but especially with CAP children, cannot be adequately developed when so many other, important areas of development have been interfered with previous to arriving at the stage of initiative vs. guilt. As the child grows, there are unfinished issues that interfere with the adequate handling of the following developmental stage. By the time this vulnerable child has reached school age the next stage, *Industry* vs. *Inferiority*, should have been entered.

However, since the child has not mastered the three previous stages, she/he is unable to deal with the major tasks of industry vs. inferiority. Children who have not mastered the first three of Erikson's stages are not ready to learn, and are prime candidates for the development of learning disabilities.[20,21] In addition, children with language disorders are also children with learning disabilities. This group of children then is vulnerable to the development of learning disabilities on two levels, linguistic and emotional.

Children who cannot learn in school are unable to develop an adequate or stable sense of competence that is the primary developmental task of the school-age child. These children tend to be seriously depressed and experience despair. They feel doomed to inadequacy and mediocrity, looking to the world as depriving them. They often exhibit inappropriate social behaviors that result in poor peer relationships. They are also ignored by their classmates and tend to be isolated within the classroom. They tend to misunderstand the communications of others, which lead them to respond inappropriately. These children are often seen as tactless, disrespectful, and/or negative, both by peers and adults. The nonprofessional adult can pick out these children as "different" from their peers.

There is a high correlation between both serious emotional difficulties and delinquency[24,25] with school failure, i.e., learning disabilities. Failure in the first major tasks of living leaves the individual vulnerable to adopting antisocial behaviors as a way of coping with their frustrations both socially and educationally. Delinquency is also a way for the individual to state that she/he experiences the environment as having let her/him down and now is going to pay society back.

Both the speech/language pathologist and the clinical child

psychologist are invested in helping children use language to express their thoughts and feelings, for according to Fraiberg,[3]

> Words substitute for an act. And this leads us into a discussion of one of the most important functions of language. Words substitute for human acts and the uniquely human achievements of control of body urges, delay, postponement, and even renunciation of gratification are very largely due to the higher mental processes that are made possible by language. The human possibility of consciously inhibiting an action and renouncing, if only temporarily, an expected satisfaction, is largely dependent upon the human faculties of judgment and reasoning, functions which are inconceivable without language. (p. 115)

According to a 1979 Carnegie Corporation[26] report, thought grows through language and conversely, language expresses thought. Without language, concepts, generalizations, and abstractions cannot be developed. Peer relationships, shared play, and fantasy do not occur, leading the child to social isolation.

The speech-language pathologist, the audiologist, and the clinical child psychologist should be committed to seeing the total child and in helping children to grow and develop to their potential. These children require all of us working together, from different professional stances, in order to serve their best interests.

4

Language Learning Disabilities Identification and Evaluation

Identification of a central auditory processing disorder is not a simple task. Often children with auditory processing problems go undetected, undiagnosed and mislabeled as emotionally impaired. The central auditory system, as noted earlier, cannot be easily evaluated because knowledge of this area is still extremely limited. In addition, traditional tests used to assess the peripheral hearing mechanism are not sensitive enough to evaluate the structurally complex higher auditory pathways.

A central auditory processing disorder has been given numerous labels depending on which professional discipline is discussing the topic. The limited interdisciplinary exchange and the confusion regarding "labels" has caused delays in the development of efficient protocols for testing children suspected of having CAP disorders. Without the collaboration of data from speech/language pathologists, audiologists, psychologists, educators, and specialists in the medical profession, it is difficult to substantiate the specific learning problems, emotional difficulties, and cognitive delays and thus provide subsequent remediation.

Parents and teachers are usually the first to present a concern regarding a child's learning. The behaviors listed below often trigger parental/teacher referrals of the child to professionals.

Children who have central auditory processing disorders (CAP) often have other associated problems such as delayed speech and language development, below grade academic achievement, hyperactivity, distractibility, short attention span,

TABLE 6

Academic difficulty.
Short attention span.
Inconsistent responses to sound.
Easily distracted by auditory and visual stimulation.
Difficulty following directions.
Difficulty recalling information obtained verbally.
Reading difficulty.
Problems with phonics.
Problems in spelling.
Poor handwriting.
Gross or fine motor coordination problems.
Poor self-image.
Difficulty understanding speech in noise.
Generalized speech and language disorders.
Significant lowering of verbal IQ.
Oversensitivity to sound.
Complaining of poor or inconsistent hearing.
Articulation difficulty.
Shyness.
Daydreams.
Impulsive behavior.
Problems making friends.
Cries easily.
Fearful of new situations.
Restless.
Worries more than others.
Denies mistakes or blames others.
Fails to finish things.
Feelings easily hurt.
Childish or immature.
Easily frustrated.
Mood swings.
Very active, always "in motion."

and learning disabilities. However, children with this disability are not a homogenous group. There is no specific grouping of behaviors that all CAP children demonstrate. Auditory processing problems may run a continuum from an attention deficit disorder to a global language problem. The listing of behaviors in Table 6 were noted in the literature and by no means are an inclusive list, but clearly demonstrate how diverse a child's behavior may be depending on the degree of the problem and length of time before evaluation and treatment. There is a close relationship between auditory perception and emotional development. If a child is unable to learn appropriately due to an inefficient auditory system, it is likely to affect her/his academic progress and thus self-image.

In order to evaluate thoroughly a child for a central auditory processing disorder, a complete case history, encompassing medical, developmental, academic, and behavioral backgrounds should precede any diagnostic procedure. It is important to specify if any prenatal problems were present such as maternal alcohol and drug ingestion, viral insult, and trauma. Birth history should be reviewed to determine if difficulties were present at birth, such as lack of oxygen to the baby, difficult delivery, or fetal distress, which places the child in a high risk category. Physical development, including auditory behavior, should be evaluated for normal milestones. A review of the child's speech and language development provides critically important information to the examiner regarding the presence of a CAP disorder. Family history of any learning, speech, or hearing disorder should also be noted and explored. Finally, academic difficulties and behavioral concerns need to be extensively reviewed and analyzed.

Of recent concern to clinicians and educators is the impact of *serous otitus media* on auditory processing and language learning. Serous otitus media is an inflammation of the membrane of the middle-ear cavity (see chapter 1) caused by a malfunction of the eustachian tube. A watery fluid is secreted by the middle ear cavity causing a hearing loss. Better known as "fluid," this asymptomatic disease is the most frequently identified cause of hearing loss in infants and young children. The incidence of otitus media in the pediatric population has been reported to be of such magnitude that it constitutes a major health problem. Ruben[1] noted that an incidence as great as 20 percent of the school-age population may demonstrate this conductive hearing loss.

Serous otitus media presents a fluctuant mild conductive hearing loss that causes a disruption in sound reception during the most critical period for language acquisition, birth to three years of age. As L. Fisch[2] so poignantly noted "the raw material of language is sound" (p. 37). An alteration in the normal reception of sound can impact on the acquisition of critical information regarding phonological, syntactical, semantic, and pragmatic parameters of language. Further, it is theorized, through research with animals, that continued deprivation of sound, as with serous otitus media, may result in permanent anatomical and physiological changes in central auditory structures that is akin to brain damage.[3,4,5]

The deleterious effects of serous otitus media on language learning and academic performance are documented in numerous studies.[6,7,8,9,10,11,12] The suggestion is also made that the effects of the learning/language problems go beyond the actual diseased state. That is, the impact of the learning/language problem created by the recurrent chronic otitus media may be irreversible. Further documentation of this was reported by Masters and Marsh.[13] In their study middle-ear pathology was found to be more prevalent in children classified as learning disabled. A later study done by Bennett et al.[14] also indicated a significantly higher incidence of middle-ear disease in learning-disabled children when compared with a normal learning group which was supported by Brandell and Seestedt.[15]

Audiologic evaluation of peripheral hearing is the first step in any assessment of a child with a learning problem. The hearing test should include an *air and bone conduction, pure tone audiogram.* In this testing the earphones are placed on the child's ears and she/he is asked to raise a hand when a tone is heard. This procedure gives the audiologist information about the degree and type of hearing loss a child may have. In addition to this procedure, *speech audiometric testing* is done to determine if a child's ability to hear and understand speech is within normal limits. This task requires the child to repeat back specific words to the examiner. This test only assesses peripheral ability and does not evaluate higher-level speech processing.

An objective, simple test designed to provide more information regarding the functioning of the middle ear system is called *impedance* or *immittance.* This test should be a routine part of any audiologic workup since it is very sensitive to identifying serous otitus media and other medically treatable middle-ear problems. This is not a test of hearing, but rather an evaluation of the stability of the middle ear (refer to figure 1). An earplug is placed in the child's ear canal and an airtight seal is created. Air pressure is varied in the ear canal producing a slightly "plugged" feeling. The response of the middle-ear system (eardrum and ossicles) to changes in pressures created by the earplug, provide the audiologist with valuable diagnostic information.

The procedures mentioned above are routine assessment techniques and can be done at any hearing clinic preferably by an audiologist certified by the American Speech Language and Hearing Association, and who is experienced in testing children.

When peripheral hearing is normal, an audiologic evaluation of central auditory processing can then be done. The basis for CAP tests were derived from extensive research in the area of human processing of sound. Normal hearing listeners are able to understand speech in the presence of background noise or even when the speech signal is distorted in some way. The repeatability of speech, or its redundancy, combined with the synthetic ability of the listener allows for understanding to occur. Filling in the "missing pieces", and deciphering a distorted message are consistent with an intact central auditory processing system. Conversely, researchers have found that individuals with confirmed central processing lesions cannot repeat back speech messages when the signal is degraded in some manner, i.e., the signal is either filtered, temporally altered, or a competing message is presented to the same ear or a competing message is presented to the opposite ear.[16,17,18] Based on the above research with adults test materials have been developed. Only recently, however, have researchers attempted to study central auditory processing in children and develop tests for use with them.[19,20]

There are few audiologic tests for evaluating central auditory processing problems in children that provide normative data. Further, these tests are applicable only after the emergence of language since the child is required to repeat stimulus items. These measures only evaluate the *functional integrity* of the auditory system. They provide limited information regarding the speech, language, or learning problem a child may have as a result of the CAP problem. None of these tests should be used in isolation to "diagnose" the presence of a CAP disorder. Only when the results of these tests are used in combination with the speech/language evaluation, psychological assessment, and teacher/parent observation should the diagnosis of central auditory processing disorder be made.

Speech/Language Evaluation

Misunderstanding and controversy exist in identifying and describing language disorders and the attendant learning disabilities that occur. There is disagreement as to which tests should be used for evaluation as well as the types of remediation that will be effective with these populations. There is also disagreement among researchers, theorists, and professionals concerning the basic problem, be it language disorder or learning disability. Researchers from various fields tend to label disabilities in terms of their discipline's definitions with which they are most familiar. For example, terms like *minimal brain dysfunction, dyslexia, specific learning disability, language disorder,* and *perceptual deficit* are just some of the terms that one often hears to describe the same phenomenon. Two terms that appear to be most effective in characterizing the child with whom we are concerned are *specific learning disability* and *language-learning disability.* A definition that most theorists agree upon include the following characteristics:

1. The child shows discrepancy between expected and actual performance.
2. There is no hearing loss, and visual acuity is normal.
3. There is no mental retardation, cultural deprivation, or severe emotional problems.
4. The disorder or disability is related to the basic learning processes.

The deficit or neurological impairment may be so subtle that it may not even be evident on neurological tests. Table 6 listed many characteristics and behaviors of children who have central auditory processing problems. We have found that children with learning disabilities often show similar characteristics. However, we cannot state that these behaviors are unequivocally experienced by all of these children. Each child must be viewed independently, for no two children are exactly alike and no two children have exactly the same type of problem.

As we stated in chapter 2, the child gradually learns language and language meanings i.e., children learn imaginative functions of sound play that then develop into rhymes that develop into stories. Halliday[21] theorizes that language occupies a key role in the social growth and learning of children. The author states that the very organization of language reflects the changing functions to which language is used from its earliest beginnings to its fully developed adult forms. The various uses of language may be seen as the child realizes and understands different intentions. However, children with language learning disabilities do not understand these different intentions, nor can they use language competently or flexibly.[22,23] These children:

1. Often have a communication style that can be labeled as egocentric. This means that it is difficult for them to understand that everyone does not think as they do. These children have problems adapting in social situations. They assume that the person to whom they are speaking, or the listener, knows the sequence they know or the events about which they are speaking.[24,25]

> For example, a six-year-old boy when telling about his summer vacation said: "And we finally got there and ate. But she told us that we were too late to see the other kids because they got tired and went home."
>
> This child is making the assumption that the listener knows exactly what he is talking about and to whom his pronouns refer. This is an example of very poor communication because the child is not sharing material clearly and has failed to take the role of the listener.

These children at the same time, do not process information well in interactions. Children with egocentric communication styles do not consider the age or background of the person to whom they are speaking. They usually give an amount of information that is inadequate to convey their communicative intent.

2. Often convey messages that are characterized by uncreative patterns using simple sentences without nuances.[26]

> An eight-year-old-boy was asked to describe an event which happened in his family. He said: "Me and my sister were making the face and my brother dropped the paint and uh, uh, Mom yelled and uh we got done and my brother cried."

Children with language deficits do not rehearse: They do not plan what they are going to say, therefore experiences and events are often not related sequentially.[27] Rather they describe things in a more freely associated manner. Sometimes this makes the message sound incoherent. Below is an example of an eleven-year-old boy who was told to explain the way in which a telephone works:

> Let's see, uh you put it by your ear and you talk into it. If someone is there, you can ask to talk to your friend. If you are not at home you have to put money in the box.

Here is another example from a ten-year-old girl who was asked to give an explanation, in sequence, of how to make pancakes. She said:

> You cook them in a pan, but first you make the batter, but first you open the box, and then set the milk in it and put syrup on them.

You will notice, especially in the last example, that there are false starts while the child is trying to decide where to begin and/or how to structure what she was going to say in her search for the right word. This is a repetitive pattern with language learning disabled children. The child does not have the ability to map or plan her/his thoughts. As a result insignificant details are added in order to gain time to organize thoughts or find the missing word. These children lose their train of thought and their listener.[28]

Carrying on a dialogue is also extremely difficult for these children.[29] They cannot maintain the interaction or make comments that are directly relevant to the conversational topic. Sometimes they will change the topic for no apparent reason because they are responding to their own associations that are not communicated to the listener. The following is an example of twelve-year-old Billy, who has difficulty maintaining a conversation. (Keep in mind that when two or more people are engaged in conversation, they are sending, receiving, clarifying, embellishing messages.)

THERAPIST:	What do you like to do for fun?
BILLY:	Make model airplanes
THERAPIST:	Tell me how you put them together.
BILLY:	It's hard.
THERAPIST:	Tell me anyway.
BILLY:	It's too hard. I can't.
THERAPIST:	Explain to me what you have to do.
BILLY:	You have to get a kit.
THERAPIST:	I have to get a kit? What do you mean?
BILLY:	You have ta git it somewheres that sell 'em.
THERAPIST:	Can you you tell me where?
BILLY:	It's better to make um from the mail.
THERAPIST:	What do you mean?
BILLY:	I can put um together better.
THERAPIST:	Do you mean you order the model kits from a catalogue?
BILLY:	Mom's got the number on her card for the mail.

It is obvious that it is not clear in Billy's mind how he can verbally describe and explain the process of putting a model plane together. In addition to carrying on a conversation, the language-learning disabled child misses out on understanding underlying messages in a conversation. Listening to the speaker, the child may have difficulty interpreting statements that may not be concrete or clear. For example:

> A teacher in an elementary school lunch room was trying to be a good model for the children and seeing the table a mess particularly where one boy sat, said to him: "Bread crumbs all over this lunch table really bothers me."

Now the teacher assumed that the boy to whom she was speaking would be able to infer the underlying meaning: next time clean up the table after you finished your lunch. The child with a language-learning disability cannot interpret that subtle message; i.e., bread crumbs all over the table really annoys me. The teacher would have to say quite directly, "The next time clean up the table after you have finished your lunch. Bread crumbs all over the table really annoys me." The child's inability to interpret the unstated subtle message causes adults to be impatient with these children.

Children with learning disabilities have poor mapping skills or planning skills that result in sharing experiences and events that are not related sequentially. They also have significant problems creating stories and fantasizing. For example, a ten year old girl was asked to make up a story based on a picture of a family having a picnic in their backyard as part of a language evaluation.

> There is a mom and dad cooking. A cat is coming in the yard. He is hungry I wonder where he's gone! There is a kid there and he can't fix anything. He liked the hamburger but she hates vegetables. The baby got sick and threw up. She spilled the pop and Dad got mad so they all stopped. But the lady next door came to see the mother and dad wasn't mad anymore. The fire was hot and they didn't have any more stuff to put on it.

We also see that deficiencies in language affect other modes of communication, such as reading and writing. Children who are language learning disabled are not comfortable with words or language because they have poor comprehension of communication. If the child cannot revise or change statements on the basis of what he or she sees and understands, or if the message is not clear, written work will be poorly constructed and difficult to understand.[28]

Tests and Testing

When children are referred to a speech pathologist for a suspected language-learning problem, the clinician must first determine whether or not a speech or language problem is present and if so, describe the problem as it is manifested. To accomplish this, there are standardized and systematic methods of testing. These tests are based on the standard of speech and language required for a particular child at their particular age. In the last two decades, an abundance of formal language tests have been developed. Some of the tests focus on the measurement of skills that are thought to be necessary for language acquisition, i.e., auditory memory, auditory perception, auditory association, etc. Some tests look at specific speech or language skills such as articulation, receptive vocabulary, expressive language, understanding syntax, still others look at use of language.

There are a number of tests that include psychodiagnostic flaws, inadequate samples, poor test reliability and many other deficiencies. Most serious are the ones that fail to demonstrate consistent validity, which refers to the degree to which a test measures what it is intended to measure. Speckman and Roth,[30] Lieberman,[32] and Michael[31] point out numerous flaws across a wide range of speech and language tests. Results from using a test instrument that was not designed with a theoretical framework, may not yield meaningful data. A clinician who uses tests that are not theoretically grounded to construct a remediation program will not meet with success. In spite of the large number of tests, there is still a need for measures to differentiate between the language of a normal child and the language of a disordered child. Assessments are also needed that will identify subtle language problems. Therefore, because of the wealth of available yet inappropriate tests there will be no list of "appropriate tests" included in this book. In addition since each child's problems are so varied, specific tests will not be recommended. Tests should only be selected on the basis of the particular needs of the child to be tested. Identifying a child that would benefit from a speech and language evaluation is the first step in this process.

The American Speech, Language, and Hearing Association (ASLHA, 1989)[32] developed a list of behaviors that may suggest a language disorder that will interfere with the ability of a child to communicate orally as well as read and write. ASLHA divided these characteristics into the elementary, junior, and senior high school levels.

Elementary School Children

Children at the elementary school level who exhibit an inability to attend to instruction will have academic difficulties. A limited vocabulary is another indicator of a possible language-learning problem also leading to academic difficulties. Trouble retrieving or knowing what word to use just adds to the problem of achievement. Difficulty with sequencing, doing manual activities or paper and pencil tasks has led to a misdiagnosis of perceptual problems. For example, these children may have difficulties following directions in proper sequence, and expressing ideas and telling stories. Events in a particular story may not be in correct order because these children also have poor short term memory. Children with language disorders also have a poor concept of the meaning of time and related temporal concepts. All these symptoms may be expressed rarely or frequently. Limited communication or difficulty in communicating with other children as well as parents and other family member may be evident. Over use of simple sentences that was described earlier, may be another characteristic. Language-learning impaired children should be observed not only on school tasks, but in social situations. Children who seem withdrawn and are frustrated with school tasks, and have a poor self-concept may indeed be candidates for a speech and language evaluation.

Adolescents

Children at the junior high and high school level may demonstrate more complex problems. Their language learning disability may not be evident to teachers and parents at lower academic levels. However, as the schoolwork increases in complexity, the child may have more problems. Children with language-learning disabilities at the junior and senior high school levels may have problems organizing and categorizing information. They are not able to identify and solve problems independently. They have trouble thinking about ideas and events that are not visual and happening in the present. Classes like history may be difficult since these children have problems relating to events that occurred in the past.

Students who have language disabilities may not understand complex sentences and words with multiple meanings.[26] They have trouble understanding main ideas. This will show up in their inability to give book reports or write a synopsis of a story. They are not able to follow a sequence of directions given only once. This interferes with test taking, homework assignments and anything that requires more than one or two specific directions.

Students with language learning disabilities can be characterized by an inability to plan and sequence their thoughts logically. They cannot sort their thoughts into grammatically correct sentences. They are also not able to give clear directions, tell coherent stories, or explain processes in detail with clarity and accuracy. These children also have trouble providing relevant and complete answers to questions.

The older child with language-learning disabilities may not have the necessary language skills to cope with situations such as applying for a job. Some mothers have reported that their children have great difficulty using the telephone to call a friend and ask them to go out especially if it is someone they don't know very well. Misinterpreting signs and labels, another characteristic that parents, teachers, and clinicians have reported, are indicators of language-learning deficits. These children also have trouble understanding humor. They don't seem to catch on to the slang and the nuances of the language of their peers. It is important for parents and teachers to be aware of these symptoms that are subtle indicators of a language-learning deficit. These children should be referred to a speech language pathologist, and psychologist.

Evaluation

Evaluation of the nature and the extent of a language problem is usually identified or defined by obtaining a sample of the child's language performance and then using standardized tests to supply additional information as to the specific area of difficulty. It is critical to keep in mind that the assessment be performed by a trained clinician and the results not determined just by scores on a battery of tests. The most useful and dependable language assessment device according to Broen and Siegel[33] is an informed knowledgeable clinician.

The child with distorted communication may call attention to her-/himself because the language is not functional or appropriate for the child's world. The clinician has to ask the question:

What is the nature of this child's dysfunctional communication? Just as therapy needs to be individualized, so does the evaluation.[28] Each individual communication behavior is measured against the clinician's understanding of good communication at the specific age and the cognitive and emotional level of the child in need of the assessment. However, all evaluation strategies should have an underlying purpose with regard and concern for the individual child as well as a conceptual model in mind.

The evaluation process should include an assessment of all language areas as described in chapter 2. These include:

Phonology—or the sound system as an organized system of sounds. This includes all the phonemes that are included in the English language. This system is usually fully developed by the time a child is eight-years old. It is necessary, in an evaluation, to determine whether or not the child has any articulation deficits.

Syntax—or the structure of the grammar of spoken and written language. It becomes the base upon which children structure their language and includes the arrangement of words within a sentence to convey meaning (sentence structure, plurality, etc.).

Semantics—or the meaning of words. This includes gestures and relationships between words as well as meaning of specific words and utterances.

Pragmatics—or the ability to use language as a tool (to make it do appropriately what we want it to do). It is related to all aspects of life and it is necessary for success in adult life. Pragmatics refers to the interpretation that the child as a speaker makes about the listener's knowledge, interest, and intent.

All these areas must be included in the evaluation, in addition to a complete assessment of receptive and expressive language, in order to get a true picture of the child's language functioning.

Receptive Language

According to Wiig and Semel,[27] Berereiter and Englemann,[23] and Simon[28] the child should be able to integrate information within and among sentences, engage in what is called verbal reasoning and evaluate whether or not a message is complete and truthful. There are five areas that should be considered in receptive evaluation.

1. Word meaning. Consider how much information has to be understood in this following sentence:[26]

> In spite of being handicapped, Dan could deftly throw the cumbersome boomerang to the interested spectator.

Wiig and Semel[27] and Simon [28] report that the student should be able to answer such questions as who was handicapped, what was cumbersome, who did the throwing, what was thrown, how was it thrown, to whom was it thrown? In addition, it would be necessary to process the introductory phrase "in spite of being handicapped." There are difficult vocabulary items such as *deftly* and *cumbersome* that need to be understood. While students might be able to process the content of the sentence if it was stated in a simpler manner, it is important to determine that these types of sentences do pose difficulty and then we need to know at what level of complexity does the student's comprehension break down.

2. Communication must be evaluated in various forms since it is not produced in isolated sentences. The student must retain and integrate sentences that are related in chunks or segments of information. Processing involves total thought. The child must compare new information with previously learned information and then evaluate whether or not the total is complete and accurate. The student must retain and integrate sentences that are related in chunks or segments of information. By having children listen to sentences and paragraphs that contain absurdities or information that is totally inaccurate we can determine whether the child is listening and evaluate inconsistencies.[28,34,35]

Comprehension evaluation needs to include observing a child's ability to synthesize clues in tasks such as in riddles or whether they can make inferences from a series of sentences going beyond the stated facts.

3. Testing receptive language will include the evaluation of the processing of technical information. This is different from processing or imitating a series of sentences. Sometimes when children are frustrated by their lack of comprehension, they

think they are not very smart. According to Ervin and Tripp[36] they may be experiencing what is termed an *overload.* The evaluation should include an observation of conditions when a student reaches a level of frustration or breakdown in other words overload.

4. Language impaired children often are prone to misunderstand information that is presented at a rapid rate. It is important to evaluate limitations on the rate of speech that can be accurately processed by these children.[37,38,39]

5. Students may not do well in environmental noise or conversations that compete with directions from teachers or other adults in their world. Many evaluations usually take place in soundproof or isolated rooms. Sometimes it may be more advantageous for evaluations to take place where conversations are occurring so that the individual's sensitivity to auditory distractions can be observed. Giving directions to students while a TV or radio is going or a conversation is taking place may provide additional information. According to Lasky and Chapandy, this represents "Real world pressure associated with language processing."[39]

Pragmatics

Diagnosis of pragmatic problems is not an exact process because there is a lack of established norms at various age levels. Assessment of pragmatics is subjective. Diagnosing these subtle problems is a clinical process and not scientific in nature. The evaluation of children's adequacy in this (pragmatic) area is probably best achieved by direct observation of them in a variety of contexts and making judgments as to the effectiveness of the communicational interaction by clinicians well versed in all aspects of development.[34] For example, the following list would be appropriate for young children at the elementary level:

1. Ask yes/no questions?
2. Ask what, where, when, why questions?
3. Establish eye contact?
4. Initiate conversation or does the child ask for help, greet people?

5. Give directions, tell jokes and play with language?
6. Open and close telephone conversations, tell stories, express needs and feelings?
7. Does the child pretend?

All these skills must be evaluated in an appropriate, meaningful way.

As we mature, our conversation becomes more sophisticated and our pragmatic abilities increase.[27,34] More competence in this area is expected of children at the junior high and high school level, so we ask other questions. Examples of these would be:

1. Does the student establish a conversational topic and make appropriate comments?
2. Does she/he terminate a topic appropriately?
3. Does she/he ask and answer questions?
4. Does she/he listen to the speaker?
5. Does the child use language appropriate to people in regard to social status, age, sex, etc.?
6. Does the child give and take directions, give cause and effect information, tell a story, disagree verbally, understand and use idioms appropriately, use language to persuade?
7. Does the child understand nonverbal messages?

All of these items should be included in a pragmatic assessment. Further assessment of the child with language-learning problems would include observations and detailed information from other professionals, including the classroom teacher, and the parents observing situations in which the child uses language appropriately and inappropriately would assist the examiner in obtaining a more inclusive picture of a child's functional language skills.

Expressive Language

In evaluating a child's expressive language there should be what Simon[40] calls "functional flexibility" or the ability to use language for various purposes in communication. She includes the following assumptions:

1. Functional language use as was stated in chapter 2, begins at a very early age when children become aware of communication functions that will satisfy their needs and their ability to control the behavior of others. Children develop strategies in interacting with different individuals within the environment, which, according to Tough,[41] are examples of "functional flexibility." This flexibility includes expressing ideas clearly and concisely, organizing messages so others can understand them, asking questions to obtain information, answering questions effectively, giving accurate directions, summarizing messages, expressing feelings to others, and performing social rituals.[42]
2. A child should possess sufficient control of syntax so that thoughts and feelings can be effectively examined. In the evaluation clinicians need to include tasks that require the individuals to organize details coherently and appropriately. For example using tasks that require the child to describe something will result in being able to look at detail. The child should be able to describe details appropriately.[43,44]
3. The expressive message that includes planning should be organized. For example, earlier "mapping" was mentioned that is similar to a road map and leads the listener to the intended message. There needs to be what Simon,[40] Johnston,[45] Westby[46] refer to as a cognitive road map or awareness. This involves the child engaging in planning tasks such as creative story telling, describing an event, or giving directions to a play or game. The child must decide how to begin, how to sequence or how to chunk segments so that the listener or the person to whom the directions are being given can follow the chronology of events so that a conclusion can be provided. There are guidelines that can be used to analyze the quality of the student's narratives and creative stories. This type of assessment will yield much information about the child's linguistic strengths and weaknesses.

Psychological Evaluation

When referrals come from speech-language clinicians and audiologists to a psychologist there is usually concern with problematic behavior and peer relationships. Central auditory processing difficulties and the more generalized language-learning disorders will lead to problems in emotional and cognitive development. These difficulties are the result of the child's inability to understand and process the auditory and language component of the environment, a skill that begins to develop with the first infant-caretaker interaction. Physicians frequently diagnose these children as suffering from an attention deficit disorder and then medicate them. Sometimes they are even diagnosed as high *functioning autistic* because of their inability to understand and possibly interact with the important people in their environments. This is a symptomatic approach to the problems CAP and language disordered children present and in no way addresses the underlying causes. Thorough evaluations medically, audiologically, linguistically, psychologically, and educationally need to be done to determine the best way(s) in which to address the problems each child tries, unsuccessfully, to deal with by her-/himself.

A medical evaluation should encompass the usual tests as well as a basic neurological screening at the yearly physical of the child. If indicated, then, further tests/evaluations of a medical nature can be ordered by the physician.

Hearing and Central Auditory Processing Evaluations are done by the audiologist. These tests have been described more fully in the preceding section. Speech and language evaluations are done by the speech and language pathologist. These assessments have also been described in the first section of this chapter.

The psychological assessment should be done by a psychologist who is well versed in evaluating children of all ages as well as knowledgeable about central auditory processing problems and language disorders. In order to obtain the fullest picture possible a wide range of tests should be used. The tests used most frequently to assess children's strengths and weaknesses include:

1. Bender-Gestalt, which gives a rough screening for neurological problems.
2. Figure Drawings, which give the evaluator a beginning sense of the issues with which the child is emotionally struggling.
3. An intelligence test appropriate to the child's age and pre-

senting problem that can give an estimate of the child's functioning level, cognitive skills, and thinking style.
4. Rorschach, which gives a picture of the emotional functioning of the child as well as the issues that may be problematic and the strengths and weaknesses, coping style, as well as the developmental issues that are being dealt with.
5. Picture story test appropriate to the age of the child as a way of understanding how the child views and experiences interpersonal interactions.
6. Achievement tests to determine the academic level of the child as well as problem areas in learning.

In addition to the above-mentioned tests, the child is being observed throughout the whole procedure to gain firsthand information regarding functioning while handling a variety of tasks and in interpersonal interaction.

Behavioral Descriptions of CAP and Language Disordered Children

Behaviorally CAP children are usually difficult to differentiate from any other child, when in a one-to-one situation. In a group they are quite distinctive and even nonprofessionals can pinpoint this child as one who is "different" from the others. An important fact is that the child behaves appropriately in one situation and not another: What does this mean? Primarily, the child has acquired some important behaviors, but, cannot always use them.

The language-disordered child, on the other hand, may be difficult to differentiate in a classroom setting, but either in a group or on a one-to-one basis stands out because of difficulties, both subtle and overt, with language and communication. Why does the language-disordered child seem to fit in the classroom and not with other situations? In the classroom, where children are expected to be quiet and unobtrusive, the language-disordered child can hide, whereas in a group setting the language difficulties can soon become apparent because of the problems in communication. However, these descriptions are rather general and with both the language and central auditory processing disordered children, just as with children in general, there is a wide variety of behaviors, functioning, and understanding.

A child with central auditory processing problems often has difficulty processing sound, and in a group situation the noise of a group can be distracting to the child so that she/he does not know to what to respond. This raises the child's anxiety level and propels her/him to action, albeit inappropriate action (the child does not understand the situation and hence responds to her/his anxiety rather than to the interpersonal situation, most often in an aggressive fashion). For example:

> The parent of six-year-old Jason consulted with a mental health professional regarding his "bizarre" behavior in the classroom. He would crawl around the floor or call out answers as well as saying all the forbidden four-letter words in his vocabulary. He was also not very welcome in the homes of children from the neighborhood and he was unable to develop any peer relationships in the classroom. The therapist went into the classroom to observe the child and found the same behaviors being displayed by Jason that the parents had described to her. She was convinced that the youngster was seriously disturbed and asked for a consultation by a psychologist. The results of the complete evaluation of Jason found him to have a poor self-image, to be quite angry with the important people in his environment because they did not understand him, to have very limited understanding of interpersonal interactions, and to be having difficulties making an appropriate identification as a male. Because of the history and the test findings a central auditory processing problem was suspected. Auditory assessment and speech-language evaluation confirmed the presence of a CAP problem. The problematic behavior in the classroom was then understood as a reaction to the noises that Jason could not process or understand. He tried to block them out through his verbal and behavioral outbursts. Therapeutic and academic interventions, taking into consideration the CAP problems quickly cleared up the inappropriate behaviors.

The child with a language disorder has difficulty in understanding sounds, words (in finding the words necessary to convey thoughts and ideas), and in understanding interpersonal communications. The anxiety that is raised interpersonally when the disability is tapped further interferes with adequate functioning and can also result in inappropriate behavior whether of an aggressive nature or withdrawal. For example:

> Eight-year-old Ryan was walking down the hall with his therapist when she met a colleague and said hello in response to his greeting. In the therapy room Ryan, who was usually responsive was very quiet and withdrawn. After about ten minutes of quiet play he asked his therapist "What did he say to you?" An astute and sensitive clinician, she told the child she and the man had just said hello to one another but that he, Ryan, was very special to her and that she liked him. The clinician was able to understand the child's unspoken, unformulated question about the importance of her relationship with her coworker and what impact that relationship had on her relationship to the boy.

It is obvious that the child had many more ideas and questions in his head than he could put into words. It was the sensitivity of the clinician that allowed her to respond to his unspoken concerns that may not have been uncovered without her attunement to the child.

Both kinds of disabled children, when their needs are not met, do not feel understood, and may well feel shamed interpersonally. Further, since the environment does not understand them, they are often responded to in an unhelpful, insensitive manner. Their inappropriate behavior to an unattuned response is often focused upon as the source of the problem Central Auditory Processing, or language is not attended to (e.g., an aggressive response to the teacher when reprimanded for hitting another child who was the original provoker and then punished for the aggressive response).

Central auditory processing and language disorder problems will manifest themselves at various levels of development.

Preschoolers

Preschoolers are rarely referred to mental health practitioners because of language, auditory processing problems but rather for behavior problems. A recent study[47] of the referrals to a child development clinic in Toronto indicated that at least 60 percent of those children referred were suffering from language and related problems rather than just the behavior problems that had been picked up by nursery/day-care personnel. The presenting complaints were:

a. Behavior problems.
b. Not paying attention.
c. Not fitting in with the group.

When these children were evaluated by the audiologist and the speech and language pathologist as well as the psychologist there was a consistent set of findings. These included:

1. Language concepts delayed, yet the children were talking about people and their environment as you would expect from a preschooler.
2. The children talked about what Mommy does, the dog does, what they want to do, etc. They had a "here and now" language that seemed intact. As long as there was something in front of them they could *see*, they could talk about it.
3. The ordering of words to make a sentence was problematic for these children as they left words out, used tenses incorrectly, and/or transposed words. They were delayed in responding to what was said or went "huh?"
4. These children did not handle each sequence of information, they did not remember all the components, they did not do it in the right order, got parts of the sequence incorrect, in other words, they misheard and misunderstood what was said to them.
5. These children did not have good problem-solving strategies nor could they talk about their needs, their frustrations were enacted in problematic behavior.

The above mentioned problems interfere with adequate cognitive and emotional/social development and eventually adequate functioning both within the family and within the peer group. How does this occur?

In the beginning, as children learn language, they begin to label objects and people in an interpersonal relationship. Within the structure of the relationship children learn how to understand facial expressions, turn taking, modulation of voice, the coordination of affect and inflection, etc. When a child has trouble processing the linguistic and auditory components of interpersonal relationships, disturbances in all areas of functioning ensue. As the child moves out into the wider environment and must learn to function with peers, the difficulties in understanding and producing language become more critical. Without adequate language children cannot develop the skills and concepts necessary to master increasingly complex cognitive, social, and emotional tasks. They may become distracted because if they do not know what to pay attention to or cannot understand what is being said they cannot learn new material and new ways of doing things. Problem-solving skills are arrested at a level of development inappropriate for age.

The list of tests previously discussed with some modifications, can be used to assess the preschool child, the school-age child, and the junior and senior high school student.

School-Age Children

A wide range of behaviors are exhibited by the school-age child with central auditory processing and language problems that could be considered problematic. This age group like their younger counterparts are often referred for behavior problems with the primary question of an attention deficit disorder with hyperactivity and learning disabilities. Many of these children are placed on medication (Ritalin or Cylert) which sometimes has an impact on the problematic behaviors. However, in most cases medication does not help the child learn any better than before (see chapter 1). Rather than prescribing medication solely on the basis of behavioral symptoms a complete evaluation of the child should be done routinely. Assessing the child can give all the clinicians involved a picture of the child as she/he sees her-/himself. Then a reasonable and considered course of remediation can then be instituted, tailored to the needs and problems of the specific child.

Junior and Senior High School Children

The problems created by central auditory processing and language problems only become intensified as the child moves into junior and senior high school where higher and more abstract (adultlike) levels of thinking and understanding are expected. It is this group of children who tend to be the high school dropouts because learning has typically resulted in failure. Teenagers with language and central auditory processing problems have been overrepresented in the group of youngsters who have been involved in the juvenile-justice system. Again, the inability to understand interpersonal interactions lead to failure both personally and interpersonally.[48,49]

5

Treatment and Intervention

A typical classroom situation creates a less than optimal listening situation for children. Background noise generated both inside the classroom by heating ducts, lighting fixtures, normal activities, etc., or outside the classroom by traffic, cafeteria, or playground can interfere significantly with a child's ability to attend, clearly discriminate speech, and thus learn. Sound levels in unoccupied classrooms have been found to exceed even recommended noise levels for understanding speech.[1,2] Thus it would seem that average sound levels found in typical classrooms with students present will interfere with auditory communication.

Background noise by itself does not produce the major concern regarding classroom acoustics. It is the difference between the primary speech signal and the extraneous background noise in the environment that causes difficulty in understanding. This is referred to as the signal to noise ratio (S/N ratio). The amount of information that is understood in a classroom will decrease as the signal-to-noise ratio decreases. A favorable signal-to-noise ratio allowing children to function effectively in a classroom has been designated at +10 to +12 dB S/N ratio,[3,4] that is, the speech signal should be 10 to 12 dB higher than the background noise. Unfortunately few existing classrooms meet this criterion. Kindergarten and elementary classrooms studied by Sanders[1] were found to vary from +1 dB to +5 dB S/N. The teacher's voice was only 1 to 5 dB over the extraneous noise present. Signal-to-noise ratio is one of the most important factors in improving speech intelligibility.[5]

When *reverberation* of sound is coupled with a high S/N ratio and speaker distance, intelligibility of speech is even more affected. Reverberation refers to a prolongation of sound similar to an echo effect. Sound is not absorbed but rather reflected back. The reverberation time in a room is most directly responsible for the quality of the listening environment.[5]

Unwanted sound is detrimental to the learning environment. When classroom noise is coupled with an auditory processing disorder, not only does a child have difficulty attending, but he/she may be unable to piece parts of an incoming message together. The pieces remain segmented and are processed in the brain in that manner. When the information is retrieved, it is often distorted and inappropriate. It is critical, therefore that any classroom therapeutic approach implemented with a central auditory processing-disordered child initially examine the classroom environment. Reducing noise and increasing the teacher's voice will maximize learning situations.

Often classroom noise can be reduced by isolating such things as defective lighting structures, broken fans, blowers in heating/cooling systems, or adding carpeting to highly reverberant areas. Additionally, classroom management and discipline can impact on noise levels. Outside noise generated by traffic, or industry for example, is not as easily isolated or dealt with. Examining the noise environment of a child is important, but having the ability to modify the noise significantly, especially when it occurs outside of the school may not be realistic.

Examining the acoustic environment of the classroom and making any modifications possible will aid all the children in that classroom in learning. Additional suggestions for enhancing the teaching environment are discussed below and can be easily integrated into any teaching style. Appendixes A and B also provide a listing of suggestions to parents and teachers.

It is important to maintain children's attention. To do so, auditory and visual distractors should be kept at a minimum. Lessons should be presented in discrete units, using simple, consistent vocabulary and in a slow delivery style. A child should be questioned often regarding material to ensure she/he is understanding the discussion. Using a child's name or a starter phrase such as "ready" prior to asking a question alerts the child and allows her/him to prepare.

Evaluation of a CAP child's seating arrangement should be done to remove her/him from distractions such as the pencil sharpener or noisy heating system. Experimentation with different seating arrangements near different classmates may prove beneficial in reducing distractions. Optimally, the child should be as close to the teacher as possible in order to receive speech at a good level.

Have the CAP-disordered child copy homework daily from the board into a notebook. Depending on the age of the child, tape-recorded class lectures can be replayed and notes reviewed at home later.

It is advisable for CAP-disordered children to review vocabulary and basic ideas re a new lesson, prior to its introduction in the class. Familiarity with new words will prepare the child for discussions.

Materials should be presented in sequential order and if possible related to the "child's world." This will aid the child in integrating the information and retaining it. Use of other modalities or *sense training* to teach particular concepts may be advisable. Experiential learning provides the CAP child with input from other senses beside the auditory.

Encourage the CAP-disordered child to be her/his own advocate and to ask for clarification or restatement of material not understood.

During quiet study times the child should be provided with an area free from visual distractions. Earplugs or *sound-attenuating earmuffs* can be used to block out extraneous noises and allow the child to concentrate.

When possible, demonstrate to the student what needs to be done. The student should be able to envision the beginning and end of a task and should be rewarded immediately at the conclusion of an assignment.

Use a general routine or schedule that a child can refer to each day. This allows the student a degree of security and prepares him for changes in tasks.

Parents need consistent input from the teacher regarding their child's progress. Follow-up on homework assignments or pretutoring lessons can be accomplished at home.

In addition to these general suggestions a regular classroom teacher may also receive specific speech and language objectives to incorporate into her/his daily teaching routines. The speech and language pathologist is a valuable part of the intervention team and should work closely with the classroom teacher.

Classroom intervention strategies discussed above, coupled with the use of *FM auditory training equipment* has been suggested for use with CAP-disordered children. These systems optimize the auditory environment by reducing the impact of background noise by increasing the speech of the teacher.

FM systems are like mini-radio stations. The teacher transmits an FM signal via a microphone attached to a transmitter to a child who wears a receiver and Walkman-style headset. The child receives minimal amplification, however the teacher's voice is received at a much louder level than background noise in the classroom. Signal to noise ratio is increased considerably. The child hears the teacher as if "she/he were talking in her/his ear." The advantage of this type of system is that it is wireless, so both teacher and child can move about freely. It can also be used outside the classroom on field trips, etc., since regular radio FM signals do not interfere with the "educationally designated" frequencies being emitted by these units. The FM systems are rechargeable and the fidelity judged to be very good. Studies using FM auditory training systems on learning disabled children demonstrated improved attending behaviors, including participation in discussions, ability to follow directions, and awareness of verbal cues.[6]

FM systems were initially used with hearing impaired children in order to give them the best possible listening situations. Their applications have expanded considerably in the past number of years to encompass children with auditory processing problems, the minimally hearing impaired, and those with hearing loss in one ear. Although these units are somewhat costly, and require the audiologist to program and maintain them, the benefits of this type of intervention with the CAP child should be considered. For example:

> Jay was referred by a psychologist for central auditory processing evaluation. Prenatal, birth, and medical history were negative except for allergies for which the child was receiving injections. Jay was experiencing academic and behavioral difficulties and had been placed part-time in an emotionally impaired classroom.

Hearing sensitivity was normal in both ears. Subsequent audiologic CAP testing indicated below normative functioning. In addition, a complete speech and langauge evaluation revealed that Jay had difficulty in the areas of processing oral directions, abstract concepts, and problems in differentiating between literal and metaphoric expressions. Latency in responses as well as re-auditorization was obvious during speech and language testing. Jay's performance on a battery of language tests supported the diagnosis of a central auditory processing disorder.

Jay's biggest problem in the classroom was inattentiveness, which therefore impacted on his reception of directions and understanding of instructional material. He was described as generally "being out of it." An FM trainer was recommended for his use on a trial basis. Teacher and parents were counseled as to care and use of the device. It was recommended that Jay use the system during all lecture and discussion periods. Additionally, sound-attenuating muffs and a study cubicle were recommended for individual work during quiet times.

Jay acclimated well to the FM system and his attention improved significantly. Jay felt somewhat self-conscious with the unit and his parents also expressed concern re his "looking different." Teacher comments, however, were positive.

The FM system is obviously the most efficient method of providing an acoustically "clean" environment for hearing. Another system, however, is available to reduce background noise and enhance teacher signal. This unit is a *sound field amplification device*. The teacher utilizes an FM microphone and transmitter that sends a signal to a receiver attached to an amplifier and speaker. The speaker may be located in the back of the classroom. This unit allows the teacher to maintain a consistent signal approximately 10 dB above the ambient noise level in a room. Children in the back of the class receive the teacher's voice as well as children in the front. Results of studies done using this method revealed significant improvement in academic achievement test scores in a group of students exposed to this application.[7]

Amplification systems offering minimal loudness but requiring the teacher to be connected to the student by a wire are also available at less cost than the two systems mentioned above. The teacher is, in effect, tied to the student via a microphone she/he is using that is plugged into an amplifying device the child wears.

These units offer good fidelity but are not designed to be worn on a daily basis. They may be useful for shorter periods of time when the teacher is working with small groups or is lecturing at a podium.

The above-described systems coupled with classroom intervention and the support services of a speech language pathologist and special educator can maximize the potential of a child with a central auditory processing problem.

Speech And Language Intervention

The authors have emphasized the significant variations in the profile of all children with language-learning deficits. Not only is there a wide variety of deficits, but research has demonstrated that a technique that appears to work well with one child does not work with another. Learning new language abilities is on a continuum that proceeds at an uneven rate. The acquisition of language abilities is on a continuum that proceeds at uneven rates. This explains, in part, why one child will benefit from an intervention method while another does not. This learning difference depends upon the profile of the child's stage of language development and the nature of the language disorder itself.[8,9,10]

Using a developmental model provides a clear focus for planning intervention. Intervention needs to be paired with functional communication (e.g., greetings and other social conventions) and compensatory strategy models (e.g., numeric devices, visual imagery). Not only must therapy facilitate language as it normally develops, but it must also consider the child's particular disability. Research is needed to explore the timing of treatment to determine if there are optimum times for providing direct treatment in relationship to maturation or growth spurts. Treatment may be more beneficial at particular times while not at others. We do know however, that the younger the child begins treatment the better the prognosis.[11] We also must work as a team to insure that the child's self-concept does not begin to interfere with the learning process. Significant problems with peer relationships and adjustment to school also will have negative effects on self-concept and language learning. We must begin to work early and consistently with the child recognizing these possibilities, so that compensating negative consequences can be addressed.

A review of research in intervention and clinical management provides the following list of assumptions that can act as a guide to speech and language pathologists and also to parents and teachers.[12]

1. Direct treatment is required for a child who is slow in one or more aspects of language development or who has specific biological or behavioral characteristics that identify her or him at risk for a delay in development. They should be referred for direct treatment.[13]
2. When treatment is provided at an early age, the better the outcome. The more people involved in intervention, the better the results.[14,15]
3. Language intervention can facilitate the child's growth of language linguistic abilities and even help him or her catch up to peers.[13]
4. Language intervention will facilitate the impaired child's linguistic performance. Without such intervention the child's potential may not be realized.[16,13]
5. Language intervention facilitates overall language development. When this happens a child is said to have learned a strategy or means of acquiring language and thus acquires new linguistic forms and functions.[17,18]

Research has not been designed to address whom and what to treat directly, how and when to treat, or for how long to treat. However, data does suggest that there are some principles for making decisions on therapy and treatment.[12] A decision as to whether a child will benefit from no treatment or direct treatment, individual treatment planned by speech/language pathologist and implemented by a parent or teacher, should be based on existing data and results from thorough evaluations. There are few guidelines regarding which children do benefit from treatment. If they are in treatment, it is sometimes difficult to know whether direct treatment or a team approach would be best. The normal developmental model, has been used, as stated previously, almost exclusively for determining which children should be enrolled in treatment.[11,19,20] The identification of a language delay using a normal developmental model only tells us that the child deviates from peers (the norm). It does not give us information on the potential for change or what type of service would be best. It is the opinion of the authors of this text based not only on research but also on their extensive clinical experience, that children who are treated with a team approach that includes teachers and parents will demonstrate more carryover into their normal environment and thus more competency in functional language use.

It is impossible to define specific objectives for treatment since children will vary not only with age, but with degree of deficit, type of deficit, prognosis, etc. General principles will be provided in this chapter regarding some existing strategies and therapeutic principles.

Thinking Skills

A language-learning disordered student is not challenged to extend her/his thinking processes. Many of the activities presented to these children involve only recalling facts stored in short-term memory, in repeating information and/or identification tasks. Current research[16] indicates that students need to be challenged into developing higher levels of thinking, especially those children who have been identified as having deficiencies in language. Wilson, Lanza, and Barton[21] have utilized Bloom's Taxonomy Classification System[22] of cognitive domain to develop a unique and creative application that is suitable for developing therapy in areas of speech-language pathology. This model is suitable for children from preschool through high school. An orderly step-by-step lesson has been designed with suggestions for the use of social studies, history, language arts, or reading. Any story, fact or fiction, is suitable if the student is interested in it. There are four basic steps that must be followed:

1. A story needs to be selected or one can be written by the student, teacher, parent, or someone who is well acquainted with the child.
2. Questions need to be asked and the plan for asking a question has to be based on Bloom's *Levels of Thinking*.[22]

3. The story must be read to the student, or if the student is able, the student should read it orally.
4. All questions must be presented orally to the student by the teacher, parent, or clinician.

Initially the student needs to be told that this is an exercise that will be enjoyable and there are no right or wrong answers. Many children with language-learning disabilities are fearful of answering questions because their responses have been wrong so often. The goal is for the students to use their thinking in new and creative ways. Bloom's Taxonomy is divided into levels of thinking, demanding increasing complexity of cognitive skills. These skills build one upon another. The example that will be presented is suitable for young children but the framework can serve as a model for students at all academic levels. (The story of "Cinderella" can be selected by the therapist.)

1. *Knowledge:* Objective—Recall facts and details from the story. How many characters are in the story? Name some of the characters in the story. What did Cinderella do? Why did she have to work so hard?

2. *Comprehension*: Objective—Understanding the story ideas. The student will understand the story ideas well enough to explain them to someone else.

   a. Tell two things you remember from the story.

   b. Tell me how the story ended.

   c. What did Cinderella do when she came home from the party?

3. *Application*: Objective—The student will describe how the story relates to the child's own life or to a situation the child has experienced.

   a. Did the story remind you of a situation that you have ever experienced? Tell me about it. One of the words in the story was *carriage*. A carriage is something people ride in. Have you ever seen a carriage or have you ever had a ride in one? Tell me about it.

4. *Analysis*: Objective—The student will take the story apart by sequencing, comparing and contrasting different parts.

a. Compare Cinderella's fairy godmother to your godmother. How is your godmother like the one in the story? How is she different from your godmother?

b. Tell something that happened at the beginning of the story, the middle of the story, and at the end. Think of another story that you may have read, such as "Snow White." Was Cinderella like Snow White? How was she like her? Think of something that might have happened when the story ended. What things could really have happened? What things were just fantasy?

5. *Synthesis*: Objective—The student will use a story idea to develop an original presentation. The child can draw a picture about a part of the story, act out the story, or write a radio or TV script of the story. The child can change the story, or change the ending, or plot. The story can be made funny or sad. This provides an opportunity for writing another story with the same theme.

6. *Evaluation*: Objective—The child will make a judgement about the story based on a particular standard. The student will be asked whether or not she or he liked the story; if not, why not. Compare the story that was read today with one that was read yesterday or last week. Ask questions. Should Cinderella be expected to do all the housework by herself?

Wilson, Lanza, and Barton[21] elaborate on this technique and suggest that objectives such as turntaking, asking and answering questions, and clarifying information can also be included. They also believe this model appears to be an excellent tool to evaluate and facilitate vocabulary development and other linguistic skills. The student practices language using materials taken from regular coursework, thus giving the curriculum material much more meaning. Children learn new facts and gain confidence allowing these skills to generalize into classroom and social settings.

Annie was a ten-year-old-girl who had been identified as having a central auditory processing problem as a result of an audiological evaluation. Her performance on a battery of language tests was just slightly below age level so that she did not qualify for special services. Annie's mother engaged the help of a speech pathologist in private practice to work with her daughter for an hour and a half each week. Annie's primary problems included an inability to follow a series of auditory directions, had trouble taking notes in class, could not do problem-solving tasks and had difficulty with reading comprehension. The therapist designed a program based on the Wilson Lanza Barton Technique. After approximately sixteen months of weekly management sessions Annie was able to develop effective learning strategies to cope with her language-learning disability. As she began to improve in academic skills, her grades and self-esteem showed a positive change.

This method is compatible with developmental theory and it is extremely effective. The child who uses this method in one situation can be helped to carry it over to another related situation. This type of activity is also well suited to group work as it allows the teacher or the clinician to observe the child interacting with her/his peers. The therapy should be based on the child's experience in real situations and group interactions. The lived experience is critical for carryover; and should be pragmatically appropriate. The experience should not violate expected social norms.

Pragmatic Therapy

There are some language deficits that appear to respond quite well to specific techniques. Management of pragmatic deficits and language problems that result from auditory processing deficits appear to benefit from the utilization of the management model formulated by Wiig and Semel.[23]

Pragmatic Therapy with Elementary School Children

Therapy for young children with pragmatic deficits should focus on repetition and reinforcement.[23] An experience-based language therapy program should be initiated in which a child takes part in actual activity. The teacher or speech-language pathologist should model the language appropriate to the activity that stimulates the child.

Presented here is an example of a pragmatic activity that may be used with elementary children in a group setting. The activity is designed to facilitate conversational skills:

> The children are presented with pictures of familiar scenes (farm, playground) or events (birthday party, eating at McDonalds) and drawing materials. Each child must describe her/his picture to the other children in the group who will then try to duplicate the descriptions. The goal is to have similar pictures among the children. Children will use language to give complete relevant directions, describe, interpret, and ask for information.

Pragmatic Therapy with Junior High School Students

Learning-disabled adolescents sometimes have subtle and often-undiagnosed language problems. Many times they are still suffering from the results of earlier language disorders that have interfered with their educational, social, and emotional growth. Junior high school students are at an age when peers become increasingly important. Youngsters with communication deficits have very little chance of being a member of a peer group, which includes being understood by the group and understanding the language of the group. They fail to comprehend the slang and idioms of their peers. Since they fail to comprehend dialogue, they become more and more reluctant to enter into conversation and fall outside their peer group. It is critical that they have exposure to group activities where they can identify and understand social cues. The activities need to be repeated through role-playing until the child feels secure in the use of the skills. Then they can use this knowledge in real-life situations appropriately.[24,25]

> Thirteen-year-old Joel upended the Sorry board angrily when he saw that he was losing the game. His psychotherapist, rather than addressing the anger that arose from Joel's low self-esteem, talked about his good strategy in playing. His anger quickly abated as Joel focused upon his game playing. Future psychotherapy sessions found him working to refine his skills, thus leading to a more positive self-concept.

Pragmatic Therapy with Senior High School Students

Senior high school students with communication problems have obviously been frustrated throughout all levels of elementary and junior high school. These students experience a low self-esteem due to repeated failure academically and socially. The students have deficits in expressive language, and may not understand the communication system or use language to do what they want it to do. These children usually feel different from their peer group and thus are unable to interact effectively. These students need both language therapy and career counseling. Psychotherapy may also provide help in resolving the social/emotional problems that occur with language-learning problems. Therapy at this level should focus on specific areas of difficulty and help the young adult understand the communication skills necessary for adult life. If these teenagers expect to communicate appropriately in adult contexts, five areas need to be emphasized:[26,27]

1. The need to be appropriate.
2. The need to be relevant.
3. The need to give sufficient information.
4. The need to be courteous.
5. The need to make statements that provide sufficient truth value.

Therapy for adolescents and children in the upper grades may use curriculum-based subjects such as social studies, history, English, etc., as the basis for treatment. Therapy for the adolescent student, whether verbal or written, is also best presented in group context for each participant has a specific role to play. They should be participants in the development of the general plan, design their own roles, and be actively involved in the discussion.[24] This will increase the skill of the students in handling not only interactions with others, interpretation of discussions, but also written language.

Rob, is a fifteen-year-old boy who is enrolled in the ninth grade in a public high school. He attends a small group classroom for civics and math and the remainder of the day is spent in a resource room. He was referred for speech-language and hearing evaluation by a clinical psychologist who had recently evaluated him. Findings of the psychological showed that he is in the average range of intelligence with performance functioning rated higher than verbal functioning. He has both long- and short-term memory deficits because of his attention deficit disorder and suspected auditory processing problems. Reading skills are poor and far below grade level. He has poor self-concept, which is, according to the psychologist, induced by his reading problem and attention deficit disorders. It resulted in maladaptive defensiveness that effects all his relationships; peers, teacher, and family. His parents were divorced when he was five and he presently lives with his mother and stepfather. He openly states that he does not get along with his stepfather and there is constant friction in the home. Results of the speech-language and hearing evaluation indicated that Rob had difficulty interpreting, recalling, and executing oral commands. He demonstrated significant difficulties with semantic relationships such as temporal and spatial concepts. When asked, "Is noon later than morning or is noon later than afternoon," he could not answer. Rob was unable to recall and reproduce sentences of varying lengths and complexity. Performance in a test of problem solving indicated language skills were not sufficient to explain inferences, and causes of events depicted in pictures. Rob was also unable to respond to negative WH questions which again indicated he was a poor problem solver and had difficulty in following verbal directions. He was generally unhappy and disliked school immensely.

During an interview with Rob and his mother, it was obvious that Rob's mother also had serious language difficulties. She was unable to follow the written directions to the clinic and as a result Rob, who did not yet have a driver's license, was forced to drive her. During the session it was discovered that they were parked illegally. Mother had to go out and move the car and in doing so broke down in tears because she had forgotten where the car was parked, and then was extremely fearful of not being able to find it again. In conversation with her, it was obvious that her language skills were extremely limited and she demonstrated many of the same problems that were bothering her son. Treatment plans for Rob included training organizational, thinking, and memory skills using Bloom's Taxonomy Classification,[21,22] which is outlined in this chapter. These strategies included verbal mediation, rehearsal skills, and visual imagery, etc., which are also described in detail in this chapter.

Along with these general recommendations some specific suggestions for facilitating language lessons in group settings were also provided. In Rob's resource room the teacher was helped to set up group situations in which the students used story segments from popular TV shows. Story-line situation dialogues and characterizations were analyzed to examine the appropriateness of actions and to explore consequential behavior. Students learned through TV characters that they could consider alternative solutions and begin to draw their own conclusions. Commericals were used to analyze their propaganda value and to teach idioms.[28]

Rob was a young man with serious semantic deficits. He had problems with peer relationships and with his family because he did not understand the subtle messages in communication. He had difficulty understanding humor and slang expressions. This was demonstrated in his inability to draw inferences and make interpretations. Rob could benefit not only from regular psychotherapy sessions with his clinical psychologist but also from group sessions in which he could interact with peers and young people his own age in structured and monitored situations with immediate correct feedback.

Therapy for Auditory Processing Deficits

Students spend many of their classroom hours listening. They listen to oral directions for written work, for reading and spelling assignments, as well as listening to new information from lectures and class discussions. Effective processing of auditory language requires the child to be able to shift and process simultaneously at different levels. Wiig and Semel[23] and Simon[29] give two general auditory processing treatment program considerations that require both classroom teacher and parents be involved to enable the child to meet with success.

1. Develop the student's awareness of her/his role as a listener and her/his responsibility for providing the speaker with feedback necessary to obtain clarification of the speaker's message. Students should be given exercises to practice language processing and evaluate whether or not the speaker has provided enough information. This is where students learn how to ask questions to obtain information and to say, "I didn't understand."

Here is an example of a teaching strategy:

> There are three books on the table. Teacher says to the child, "Give me the book." The child replies by handing the teacher all of the books. Teacher, "No, I said give me the book." The child then says "But you didn't tell me which one." Teacher responds, "That's right, I gave you poor directions. What questions should you ask me?"[29]

This type of therapy encourages interactive skills. It helps the student to learn for example that teachers are not perfect, and that teachers and parents sometimes do not provide sufficient information for a student to complete assigned tasks successfully. Before assuming what an individual means, the student should be able to clarify what is understood and what is not understood.

2. A discussion group can be organized. Simon[30] uses a program to develop critical thinking and language processing along with discussion skills. Many of these programs are available commercially. Children then listen to comments of others, solve problems, and discuss them. Here would be an example:

> Mary's father has a big brand-new car.
> Rich people drive new cars.
> Conclusion: Mary is rich.

The students then have to consider the accuracy of the statements. Do all or only rich people drive new cars? Is Mary rich? Then they can take the validity of this conclusion, make decisions, and isolate particular factors. Meanwhile they are interacting within the group. These types of exercises may not be effective when working with children who have semantic deficits, but are effective with central auditory processing problems. For example:

> Carrie is a nine-year-and-eight-month-old girl. She was seen by a clinical psychologist through a referral from her audiologist. Her parents described Carrie as having a hard time saying what she wants to say and not always making sense. They reported that she has a difficult time functioning under pressure. However, when

she is relaxed her mother stated that "words roll right out of her mouth." Carrie has a hard time in Math and Reading. She has a history of middle-ear problems and a severe hearing loss in one ear. It was suspected by the audiologist that she also has an auditory processing deficit but because of the hearing loss CAP testing could not be done.

She was referred by the audiologist to a speech pathologist. Testing was done and results were interpreted as not indicating significant problems. She was then referred for a second opinion. This speech pathologist used a battery of tests appropriate to the presenting problems that indicated numerous difficulties in almost all aspects of language, especially in the semantic area. Carrie had serious difficulties executing verbal commands and as they became more complex was unable to complete them. Problem-solving skills indicated some serious deficits. Her scores ranged from eight years (which is almost a one year eight month delay) down to six years ten months. Sequencing in general along with following oral directions again demonstrated serious problems.

However, it was recommended that she receive some type of intervention from the school on the basis of her test scores. Because she did not meet the criteria or determination in the Special Education law, Carrie was not eligible for services from a speech pathologist.

Carrie's teacher agreed to work with her in the classroom. Some of the recommended treatment activities involved training Carrie to see how things are alike and different. It was suggested that Carrie begin to see how individual words and objects can be viewed in more than one way. Games such as Twenty Questions would be helpful.

It was also recommended that Carrie be encouraged to describe what she is doing and what she observes, to learn verbs. In other words, making instruction active rather than passive. She was encouraged to listen to and retell stories that would help her observe and describe what was happening in her environment. Role-playing is also beneficial for a child with these types of deficits.

Talking about important and not important items and events would also be helpful for her. She should be encouraged to answer who, what, where, why, and how questions about events happening in her world. This will help her to recognize that there is more to a word than just a name and a function. Guessing games would also be helpful.

In discussing Carrie's problem with her parents it was obvious that her mother also had similar problems. She herself admitted to having academic problems. She has found it very difficult to help Carrie with her homework. Since Carrie's mother has a similar disability she was encouraged to be supportive and to help build Carrie's self-esteem but to withdraw from directly helping her with her lessons. The aid of a tutor was encouraged. It was also explained that, since Carrie would be having additional help in school, Mother would help her most by encouraging her. It is not unusual to find that when children have serious reading and language deficits that a parent or a sibling may be similarly identified.

Language and Reading Skills

It has been established that there is a strong relationship among oral language, auditory processing and reading skills.[31,32,33] Therefore, children who are experiencing language deficiencies need programming prior to, or at least along with, reading instruction. They must be aware of how they can map their own perceptions and thoughts before interpreting the perceptions and thoughts of others. O'Brien[33] discusses problems centered on reading as a method of combining observation, listening, speaking, and reading to focus on the environment. For example, a very individualized approach can serve as a bridge between a child's out-of-school experience and in-school experience. Halliday[34] suggests that we have to build up an image of language that enables us to look at the way people actually do communicate with each other and how they are exchanging meanings and interacting. If the reading and writing are unrelated to what the child experiences, the demands for reading-writing will make very little sense to her/him. These two activities should not seem like meaningless exercises. They should make sense and match the child's experience of language. She/he should see reading and writing as a means of enlarging experiences and not as totally isolated exercises.

> "I can read what I can write and what others have written for me to read."[35]

The meaning of this phrase by VanAllen and VanAllen[35] refers to having a child tell a story about her/his experiences or a set of sequential pictures. The clinician asks questions, elicits various linguistic constructions.[29] For example:

CHILD: A little girl is lost.
CLINICIAN: Where?
CHILD: In the park.
CLINICIAN: Is it an amusement park or one with trees and flowers?
CHILD: Amusement park.

As the story is being told it is embellished by details the clinician adds so the child can enrich her/his story. The child can then be asked to read the story. Even children who cannot read textbooks will be able to read the printed words just as they were dictated. These techniques eliminate the mystery of the written word and draw a connection for the child between the spoken and printed word. For some older more advanced children the clinician may ask the student to tell a sequential story in a particular tense. For example:

CLINICIAN: The girl got lost in December during a snow storm. Tell me what happened.

After the student tells the story and the clinician has recorded it, it can be analyzed for past tense cues, ed markers, past-tense verbs. Researchers[17,23,28] have said that ability to analyze the structure of written language helps to aid comprehension. By utilizing these procedures the teacher and clinician are working on three or four communication areas simultaneously. As children speak, listen, read, and write, all these components form an interacting network. The analysis and synthesis of cues are constantly occurring. In order for a child to be a competent communicator all the facets of this communication network must be working and interacting. The child's communication self-concept can be improved if she or he feels comfortable with the communication system. The teachers should analyze the communication situation before adapting materials and instructions.[28] This will enhance rather than frustrate the child.[23,36]

Jimmy, a second grader had a difficult time with all academic work especially reading. He was receiving remedial reading but was described by the teacher as not responding to any type of intervention or tutoring. Jimmy was also reported to be extremely distractible in the classroom.

A central auditory processing battery indicated hearing within normal limits. An examination of the CAP battery suggested no significant CAP problems. However, the clinical assessment done by the audiologist based on the child's history and his behavior in the testing situation suggested problems irrespective of the test findings. Therefore she referred him for evaluation by a speech pathologist. The results of this language testing indicated normal language comprehension. However, Jimmy demonstrated difficulties carrying out complex commands. He also had problems in differentiating essential from nonessential parts and purposes of various items. He did not appear to understand attributes and could not generalize from previous experiences. For example, when Jimmy was asked to tell how something felt or tasted, or what it was made of or what shape it was, he was unable not only to understand the question, but to retrieve the word that described the object, and then express the words out loud. He could not distinguish between physical and sensory features. This limited the amount of information that he understood in order to fully comprehend a particular concept. He had problems with detail and could not detect key features in words and messages.

Treatment recommendations for Jimmy stressed that he be encouraged to describe things that he liked, wanted, or lost. Through sensory tasks he should learn to share how things feel, taste, sound, smell. Guessing games using blindfolds or mystery bags may be helpful to improve his ability to describe things of different textures, shapes, and sizes. It was recommended that Jimmy be encouraged to describe important and nonimportant parts of objects. Jimmy needs to learn how to compare and contrast by identifying items that have certain characteristics: for example, things that are round, things that are red, things that are furry, etc. He should also learn to describe how things are different. For example, both a bird and a plane have wings but a bird is small and a plane is big.

Jimmy may also benefit from learning to define words. Even the words that he already knows can be good training for defining skills. Anwering who, what, when, where, and how questions about an object and people will help Jimmy learn that there is more to a word than just its name. Dictionary games can help faciltiate definition skills.

He should be encouraged to dictate from his own real-life

experiences those things that are interesting to him. The teacher can then write, from dictation, exactly the way Jimmy talks. Jimmy can watch the teacher write the symbols that code the words that he has verbally produced. This approach implements the principles that:

1. Words need to be understood in spoken form before they are presented in written form.[17]
2. Content should stimulate real-life situations as closely as possible.[18]
3. Language is something that a child understands and produces before she/he reads and writes it.[39]

There are a number of activites that can also help Jimmy in the classroom. He could accumulate a sight word vocabulary by labeling tools of daily activies; for example, toy box, pencils, crayons. Sight words can be learned by using words that serve as directives. For example, watch the fish, find the book, paint here.

Jimmy may also benefit from tactile (touch) experiences to reinforce kinesthetic discrimination. The teacher can elicit a response from him concerning drawing, such as the drawing of a car or a truck. The word truck can be written on the board and then Jimmy will trace each letter as he repeats the words. Trays of colored salt can also help him to copy and trace words for tactile experiences.

Strategies to Train Memory Skills

A set of strategies designed to facilitate memory skills was tested by Lasky.[40] This model encompasses many of the techniques mentioned in other methods. This methodology can be helpful for children as well as adults who have been identified as language-learning disabled.

1. *Verbal Mediation*—This is a technique for facilitating an impression and comprehension in problem solving tasks. Self-talk, explaining or instructing occurs. Training verbal mediation skills can be carried out by having the student verbally describe the steps which must be done in order to complete a specific task. The student is required to perform or follow each of his/her own directions. This can be done at home and

during study periods in school. The student is required to mediate verbally or verbally work through logical steps to solve a particular problem.[41,42]

2. *Rehearsal*—This consists of repeating an address, zip code number, or lists of various items. Language-learning disabled students generally do not use active rehearsal techniques. These techniques require the individual to repeat aloud, then silently by rehearsing and planning a task or assignment. In order to learn these techniques, the student repeats the task aloud, and then silently. They rehearse and plan particular tasks and assignments in this manner.[41]
3. *Paraphrasing*—This is not verbatim imitation, but is dependent upon auditory processing skills. The task is presented using the student's own words and integrated with information the student already knows. The message given by a teacher or parent is translated by the student. This technique would have to be done carefully and tactfully so as not to embarrass the student or call undue attention to her/him. This can be done both formally and informally.[40]
4. *Visual Imagery*—This involves having the student represent a mental picture through drawing or speaking. The student can be encouraged to "imagine" and then begin to focus on a specific item. This strategy facilitates auditory memory.[40]
5. *Analysis of Key Words and Networking*—The student can identify new words or concepts and then attempts to relate them to familiar ones. This would involve elaborating or building from old ideas (assimilation and accommodation) concepts. Comprehension is facilitated by the teacher's presentation of an outline listing major topics before a lesson is given and then again afterwards. This helps the child learn how to structure material and organize it.[43]
6. *A Systematic Retrieval Strategy*—This technique helps retrieve ideas from memory. Identifying main themes from stories and contextual situations and presenting ideas in a sequential, systematic way will facilitate word retrieval. Teaching to ask questions, such as: "Why is this"? and then begin to elaborate also enhances the development of strategies.[43,44,45]

Psychological Treatment

Children of all ages can compare the toys they have with the possessions of others and conclude that they do not have the same items as another child. This ability is also used when comparing ability, knowledge, and skills. A lack of skill(s) has a deleterious impact on the self-esteem and sense of competence of the child. Lichtenberg[46] has suggested that the competence and the pleasure that is derived from successfully completing tasks is the foundation for positive self-feeling. The language and central auditory processing-disordered child cannot develop feelings of mastery and competence due to her or his disabilities and the interpersonally disruptive nature of the disorders.

At a time when children are separating from parents and trying to develop an adequate sense of who they are and what they can and cannot accomplish with their current skills they still need adult help. They can become stuck at any stage of development. However, most of the time they seem unable to work through the stage of Autonomy vs. Shame and Doubt or the state of Initiative vs. Guilt. In addition to being unable to develop a sense of competence they do not make important identifications with the same-sexed parent and other important idols that are so necessary for mature functioning. They are frustrated by their difficulties in both understanding the linguistic environment, with all that entails, and their inability to obtain understanding and sensitivity from that same environment. The linguistic disability results in either interpersonal withdrawal or aggressive acting out (they become behavior problems in their classroom and at home). Problematic behavior can include:

a. Distracting others.
b. Becoming defiant when they do not understand what is going on or when they cannot follow through successfully at a task.
c. Interfering with the activities of peers, engendering their anger.
d. Aggressively interacting with both children and adults.

These behaviors lead to our assessment of emotional problems. These unacceptable behaviors are born out of the child's frustration in understanding and dealing with age-appropriate tasks. Cognitively there are also difficulties because those very experiences needed for growth in this area are interfered with because of the auditory processing and language difficulties, limited experiences, and the gradually developing emotional problems. Psychotherapy is not the only answer to this problem, but therapeutic intervention is warranted. The child needs help in learning how to listen and gain information from the auditory environment, as well as help in developing appropriate language. Here, an audiologist who is familiar with central auditory processing and a speech-langauge clinician who is familiar with language problems would be good resources to call upon. A psychotherapist, who can help all members of the family cope with the problems created by the disability, would also be helpful. The family will need help in structuring the environment for the child and finding ways of teaching information directly, which most of us pick up incidently in the course of living and interacting. The feelings of the parents and the other children in the family that are generated by the problems of the disordered child also need to be dealt with. Psychotherapy sessions for the other members of the family could be very helpful. As the family is enabled to help the handicapped child develop coping strategies to deal with the auditory and language environments, the problematic behaviors should begin to dissipate. However, the resulting changes that occur in child rearing-practices require a great investment of time and attention that can potentially become wearing. Parents need help in dealing with these added stresses and strains both in the family and marital relationships.

Psychological assessments[28] of children with central auditory processing and language problems have indicated, that as a group these children:

a. Pay little attention to details in the environment and in fact focus on global, generalized impressions typical of preschoolers. This characteristic reflects the emotional and cognitive arrests seen as a consequence of central auditory processing and language problems.
b. Deal with feelings of incompetence and inadequacy by

personality constriction. In other words they function in a small circumscribed range where they can be sure of their ability to cope with things and where they will not wind up feeling inconsequential or incompetent.

c. Do not think very highly of themselves and in fact they feel very unimportant. They do not take good care of themselves and may very well place themselves in situations of danger as they just "don't care."
d. Approach problem solving rigidly and actively. They must do something: They cannot sit back and reflect on alternative approaches. For them there is only one way.
e. Are quite responsive to feelings, both their own and those of others in the environment. This makes them prone to react immediately and often inappropriately. They are very anxious and have to do something to get rid of the feelings because they have not learned how to deal with affect.

As a group, these children tend to be depressed and passive, underneath the behavior problems. The passivity is in terms of their deep sense of helplessness, incompetence, and ineffectiveness. Given the nature of the problems, their emotional and cognitive arrest and their general sense of dysphoria, psychotherapy is usually recommended. However, change and growth are quite slow and the therapy is protracted because the central auditory processing and language problems also make the therapeutic process difficult. For example:

> After about a year of treatment with his third therapist, eleven-year-old John, now off Ritalin for some three months, told his therapist she was wrong about an idea she had expressed. She commented that he had hurt her feelings by telling her she was wrong. John seemed quite surprised and apologized, stating that he had not meant to hurt her feelings. The therapist used this opportunity to suggest that if he inadvertently hurt her feelings then he must do something similar with the kids (an experience in generalization) in his classroom, which could be one of the reasons that they give him such a hard time in class (cause-effect relationship). When he agreed that that might be the case, his therapist was then able to suggest that maybe she could help him understand what happens when he is with peers that causes him so much trouble (opportunity to learn control and to function

competently). For the first time, he perked up and seemed eager to attack this aspect of his interpersonal problems.

Parental and school involvement is also quite important because these children need educational as well as interpersonal help. A therapeutic peer group in the schools can help these children learn how they impact on their peers and hopefully learn alternative ways of interacting. Processing interactions within the group in terms of sequencing, cause-effect relationships, and putting thought and feelings into words can be focused upon. In addition, special learning techniques can be instituted.

Sutton-Smith and Avedon[47] reported on a study of the differences between those children who consistently won at tic-tac-toe and those who consistently lost. They found that those children who won were better at arithmetic, could persevere at intellectual tasks, and could make rapid decisions. Those children who consistently lost were more dependent upon teachers and parents, and more conventional intellectually. These researchers came to the conclusion that there are important relationships between skills learned in games and other aspects of personality and cognitive functioning. Games designed to help these CAP and language-learning disordered children grow cognitively and learn in the classroom would be of help. Some of these games could also be used in the home for further enhancement of the growth process. There are any number of books describing a wide variety of games that can be used. Choosing the most appropriate ones to meet the needs of the particular child is the issue.

Many language- and CAP-disordered children present problems in organizing the visual-perceptual field. Activities/games that can be used for remediation include:

- Mazes, connect the dots (using both letters and numbers for planning and sequencing).
- Design creation from a model using blocks of different sizes, shapes and thicknesses (learning of shapes, numbers/counting, size and comparison, perspective).
- Playing board games for counting, following directions and developing strategies (Sorry, Chutes and Ladders).

- Dominoes, Fan-Tan, and Casino (matching and sequencing games).

Adult help will be needed for a while to provide the internal step-by-step monitoring of the game-playing process that these children cannot provide for themselves. In other words, the adult must talk the child through the game, step by step. As the child can begin to use the process by her-/himself, the adult can phase out these aids, while at the same time can draw the child's attention to how much more she/he is doing now for her-/himself, and the pride that the child must be experiencing in doing such a good job. One further step needs to be instituted with this form of learning. This includes helping the child generalize the strategies learned in the games to other areas of functioning. For example:

> Seven-year-old Sid is one of a set of identical twins who suffered from aseptic meningitis when he was about six weeks of age. In spite of being a twin he was a full term baby weighing seven pounds one ounce. Subsequent to the meningitis his development was unremarkable, except for frequent ear infections present from five months of age and the delay in development of language that the parents attributed to being a twin, a readily understandable assumption. However, when neither twin was talking adequately by the time they were four the parents contacted a clinical child psychologist. They got opinions from a wide variety of professionals who suggested that they were overinvolved parents (professionals themselves) and to let the boys alone to grow out of their problems. After taking a history the psychologist suggested a complete speech-language and audiological assessment of both youngsters. The report from the speech-language pathologist indicated that Sid had a moderate amount of articulation dysfunction, age-appropriate auditory attention, recognition, comprehension, and memory. Further, he had good integration for one-part commands even though he often needed two trials to complete tasks. Expressive language functioning indicated good word retrieval; however, function words were omitted. Story sequencing, formulation skills, general story descriptions and general descriptive abilities were felt to be reduced. The speech-language pathologist concluded that Sid had expressive language dysfunction and a receptive language weakness that required a minimum of two half-hour individual, intensive, speech-language remediation.

Three years after the evaluation the parents requested psychological assistance as the child was in constant conflict with his father, seemed to be reluctant to try new activities, and was generally unhappy. Furthermore, he seemed to become quite rigid at times and could not let go of an approach, an idea or a particular manner of functioning. A psychological assessment found Sid to be functioning at a slightly delayed developmental level, but nevertheless was progressing rather than being stuck on a particular developmental task. Rather than psychotherapy, a cognitively oriented program one half-hour per week was designed to reduce rigidity and increase flexibility in his approach to problem solving. The tasks used with Sid (described above) included creating designs to a definite and then an indefinite model with blocks; both cubes and parquetry. This activity was used to help Sid organize the perceptual field, learn a right-left orientation for reading readiness, learn how to rotate blocks to complete a design for a more flexible approach and to feel successful. Once Sid could master these tasks with some pride and proficiency, maze tracing, matching activities, and creation of the same designs with a variety of shapes were instituted. Throughout the sessions he was quite proud of his accomplishments. At the beginning of a new activity the therapist would process the steps for him aloud, then request that he tell her what the next step was in the process. Finally, he was able to accomplish the task without any intervention. As he became more comfortable with the activities he could currently handle, more complex thinking tasks were instituted.

Again, at first the adult must make the connections for the child and as the child learns to make those connections for her-/himself the adult can withdraw the help while supporting the results.

Games in other cognitive areas can be used as well but must be instituted sequentially, meeting the needs of the child at all times. Hide-and-seek can be used to train listening skills by having children hide and make as much noise as possible so that the CAP child must pay attention to where the noise is coming from. Then she/he must locate the hiding places of the other children. The children can be asked to be as quiet as mice to push the CAP child to listen very carefully for subtle auditory cues. Number facts can also be built into the game by having the child who is "IT" count by fives, threes, fours, etc. Blindman's buff and alternative hide-and-seek games can also be used in a similar manner.

Games for children with motor and eye-hand coordination problems would include clapping games with chants, and rope jumping and their chants. Hopscotch, skully, immies, etc., are other games that enable the child to practice eye-hand coordination. Learning about right-left is embodied in the circle song-game "Here We Go Looby Loo" while finding out about one's body can be accomplished with the following chant/activity:

If I move one finger (right hand in fist, free forefinger and wiggle)
And wiggle my thumb (keep fist, wiggle right thumb)
I have two fingers moving (right thumb and forefinger wiggle)
By gum! (clap twice)
By gum! (nod twice)

If I move two fingers (wiggle both forefingers, rest of hand in fist)
And wiggle both thumbs (wiggle both thumbs)
I have four fingers moving (wiggle both thumbs and both forefingers)
By gum! (clap twice)
By gum! (nod twice)

If I move four fingers (wiggle four fingers of right hand)
And wiggle my thumb (wiggle right thumb)
I have five fingers moving (wiggle all five fingers of right hand)
By gum! (clap twice)
By gum! (nod twice)

If I move eight fingers (wiggle four fingers on each hand)
And wiggle both thumbs (wiggle both thumbs)
I have ten fingers moving (wiggle all fingers on both hands)
By gum! (clap twice)
By gum! (nod twice)

If I move both arms (move both arms, hands in fists)
And I wiggle my thumbs (wiggle both thumbs)
I have arms and thumbs moving (move both arms and wiggle both thumbs)
By gum! (clap twice)
By gum! (nod twice)

If I move both feet (shuffle with both feet)
And wiggle my thumbs (wiggle both thumbs)

I have feet and thumbs moving (move feet and wiggle thumbs at the same time)
By gum! (clap twice)
By gum! (nod twice)

If I stand and sit (stand up, sit down)
And wiggle my thumbs (wiggle thumbs)
I'll get awful tired (no movement)
And I'll quit; by gum! (two big claps)

It might be helpful to look at the age, emotional and linguistic level of the child in conjunction with the types of games most appropriate to meet the child's needs.

Four-Year-Olds

Children at this age level enjoy physical activity using large muscles, e.g., jumping, climbing, and running. Balancing on narrow ledges is also of great interest and suggests a beginning trend towards the use of finer motor control. Towards this end, painting, coloring with crayons, and making things with clay and Play-doh become important.

Five-Year-Olds

Five-year-olds can hop, skip, and maintain balance on one leg yet prefer to do what is known and familiar. Routines are important now. Skipping games, kick ball, and simple rope games with chants are special favorites. Dramatic singing games such as "Here We Go Round the Mulberry Bush," "Sing a Song of Six Pence," and "Bluebird Through My Window" often become important activities as do cutting and pasting.

Six-Year-Olds

At six, the child cannot remain part of a group for long periods of time. Group and individual games need to be interspersed. Action games such as "Looby Loo" and other such movement games along with relay races and circle games will meet the needs of the child at this age.

Seven-Year-Olds

Seven-year-olds can stick with activities for longer periods of time than they have ever done before. Simple board and card games can be introduced as can group games such as hopscotch, skully, and marble activities.

Eight-Year-Olds

There is a beginning interest in games with very specific rules. However, these children have a high energy level that necessitates active games and game playing. Tags of all kinds are important, hide-and-seek, sardines, rope jumping and dodgeball are all good games for the eight-year-old.

Nine- through Twelve-Year-Olds

This age group is interested in developing individual skills, especially for use in group and team sports. This interest functions to help the child test her/his abilities against those of other children. Team sports, gymnastics and stunts are important for this age group.

All of the games described throughout this section teach children a wide variety of skills necessary for adequate emotional, social, and cognitive development and can be used with the CAP- and language-handicapped child to enhance his or her functioning in all areas.

School Recommendations

1. Consider classroom acoustics and sources of low, constant sounds, e.g., buzzing neon lights, and keep these children away from them.
2. Looking and listening are important activities to coordinate-focus the child on both.
3. Gain the child's attention by calling her/his name or touching her/him before giving instructions.
4. Check the child's comprehension through questioning to make she/he is understanding/following what is going on.
5. Encourage the child to rephrase and restate what she/he has heard-the teacher should rephrase and restate her/his state-

ments in simpler grammar to enable the child to process what has been heard.
6. Give the child the chance to repeat statements and or instructions to themselves-this provides the child the time lag needed to adequately process what is being said.
7. Keep instructions brief and to the point.
8. Use visual aides whenever and wherever possible.
9. Children with handicaps fatigue more readily than other children and may not attend over a long period of time because of the continuous strain resulting from efforts to keep up and compete in classroom. Provide short, intensive periods of instructions with breaks so that the child can move around.
10. Limit the amount of review or homework the child must deal with on any one day.

School needs to become a place where the child can test her-/himself and begin to develop a good sense of strengths and weaknesses, competencies and incompetencies. Altering the classroom in the ways suggested above will help all the children in the long run and interrupt the ever-downward spiral of poor academic performance and achievement in these language-learning, auditory processing-disabled youngsters.

Home and family can use some of the recommendations made for the school. A fuller treatment of the family and family issues will be found in the following chapter. However, parents can help structure the family environment to maximize cooperative interactions while carefully explaining the world to the child.

Family Recommendations

1. Be consistent in rules and discipline.
2. Avoid constant negative approaches.
3. Demonstrate new or difficult tasks.
4. Use visual cues with verbalizations.
5. Ask the child to do one thing at a time.
6. Explain carefully all experiences the child has or has encountered as an on-looker.
7. Keep auditory stimulation to a minimum.

At all times the environment needs to be free from distractions so that the child can focus upon what you, the adults, are trying to communicate. When there are distractions the child should be helped to understand what is the distractor and to what she/he needs to pay attention.

Psychotherapy with children during the school years has been done in a variety of ways, e.g., psychoanalysis, behavior modification, cognitive-behavior therapy, theraplay, and play therapy, etc. An argument can be made for psychotherapy in a play modality for all children, but especially for the language-learning disabled youngster.

Play allows this youngster an opportunity to express her/his concerns by playing them out symbolically for the therapist to view, understand, put into words, and then respond to verbally for the child. Children, because they haven't reached the stage of formal operations or more adultlike thinking, generally cannot verbalize their fears, worries, and concerns as the adult can. The language-learning disabled youngster is even more handicapped in this regard because cognitive structures that would lend cohesion and logical verbal structure to her/his communication is missing from the youngster's usual style of functioning. Playing out these worries and concerns via toys allows the child to communicate much more then she/he could verbally. The therapist can then put into words the concerns of the child providing her/him with a sense that there is someone who understands.

Verbal response to a linguistically handicapped child presents a therapeutic problem requiring simplification of language to match the comprehension level of the child. At the same time it provides the child with a language/communication model that will enhance and encourage the child to practice linguistic and cognitive skills. Nevertheless, therapy in a play modality and speech-language therapy have similar goals—the enhancement of language, cognition, and emotional growth.

Treatment of the social, emotional, and cognitive problems of the junior and senior high school student need to take the particular issues of early and late adolescence into consideration. For this age group this means being just like peers. Working with a handicapped teenager under this condition tries the skills of all professionals involved.

Since pulling a youngster out of class for special services automatically makes her/him different and a potential object of ridicule, whole class or out-of-school treatment would be the way to deal with the specific handicap. Emotional and social problems and worries are of special concern for all adolescents, not only the handicapped youngster. Class discussions can be used to help the youngsters understand interactions as well as alternative ways of handling a wide variety of issues. Group discussions designed by teachers and therapists can be structured so that all youngsters must participate. Previously prepared position statements and preassigned roles for role-playing can be the vehicles for discussions.

A remediation program called Instrumental Enrichment could be used as a model for the cognitive development of the whole class, but specifically with the language-learning handicapped youngster. This program was devised by an Israeli cognitive psychologist, Reuven Feuerstein[48] and was designed to foster adequate cognitive development through mediated learning experiences. It is a three-year program that aims to help youngsters develop clear perceptions, organize space, develop ideas of conservation and constancy, develop precision and accuracy, restrain impulsivity, and eliminate trial-and-error behavior.

This program lists many behaviors seen as arising from the lack of mediated cognitive experiences. The same difficulties are seen in hearing-impaired children as well as with language-learning handicapped youngsters of all ages. These problems include:

- Giving up too soon.
- Limited remembering from day-to-day, limited retention.
- Lack of relationships between ideas and experiences.
- Limited problem solving strategies.
- Lack of curiosity.
- Egocentric thinking.
- No or limited value placed on learning.
- Inability to notice discrepancies, don't compare.
- Missing cause-effect relationships.
- Problems in expressing ideas.
- Lack of problem solving strategies.
- Missing organizational skills.

According to Feuerstein[48,49] underlying these thinking processes is a passive approach to the environment, a recent finding[31] with learning-disabled children in general. Cognitive deficiencies are due to a lack of instruction about the interactions with the environment rather than a lack of interaction with it. In other words, there have not been adequate meditated experiences, which are crucially necessary for the language-learning handicapped child. For Feuerstein the actual content of the experience is not important, rather importance is dependent upon "the extent to which the experience provides insight into the thinking process"(p. 68). Meditated experiences are provided because the therapist "constantly intervenes, makes remarks, requires and gives explanations whenever and wherever they are necessary, asks for repetition, sums up experiences, anticipates difficulties and warns the child about them, and creates reflective, insightful thinking" (p. 64). The Instrumental Enrichment program is designed to provide "problem-solving tasks, strategies for individual mediation, and discussions for insight to correct specific deficient cognitive functions and provide the prerequisites for learning. Among its many objectives are the arousal of motivation and insight, creation of good work habits, and methods of gathering and elaborating information. The program's aim is to render the individual able to perform as an independent learner by providing him or her with the concepts, skills, strategies and techniques necessary."

Psychotherapy with junior high school youngsters is not often recommended as they have a great deal of difficulty sustaining an adult-style therapy session where talking is the major mode of communication. This modality would be especially difficult for the language-learning handicapped youngster. Family therapy is the treatment of choice. However, for the language-learning disabled child the verbal interchanges may be overwhelming. Small group (four to five children at the maximum) therapy that is videotaped would be ideal. Interactions between children and adults would be taped so that they can be played back and discussed, enabling the youngster to develop understanding of his/her interpersonal functioning and its consequence.

Small therapy groups as suggested for the junior high school student can also be used for the senior high school student. However, the teenager at this age level is more able to sustain a usual verbal therapy session. Given that psychotherapy is a verbal modality this form of remediation taps into the disability, making this process a longer and more difficult one than would be otherwise, albeit a helpful one.

6

Families

Whenever a child is a member of a family, stresses of all varieties inevitably impact upon the marriage and the marital couple. These stresses are exceptionally hard when there is a handicapped child in the family.

When a child, especially a first child, is expected, dreams and fantasies are spun by the expectant parent, grandparents, and other relatives and friends. It is difficult enough when the new baby does not meet the expectations that have been generated about it, but it is even worse when a handicapped child is born. However, in both circumstances the parents must come to grips with the discrepancies between the fantasied baby and the real baby. Dealing with the "reality" involves a mourning process. The dreams that have been spun are altered or die, and are replaced by those hopes that better reflect the parents growing understanding of their child.

This mourning process[1] that enables the parents to separate from their dreams and hopes for the child includes:

a. DENIAL: a way of dealing with an uncomfortable and painful situation and helps the parents buffer themselves against uncomfortable information. It helps the person to buy time to find the inner strength and external supports to deal with the perceived loss.
b. ANGER: comes out of the question "why me (us)?" and is usually directed outward, against anyone and anything that gets in the way.
c. ANXIETY: helps to mobilize the person so she or he can

deal with the changes necessary to cope with the new situation.

d. DEPRESSION/GUILT: is a reaction to the sense of loss of hope and feelings of responsibility for causing the handicap.
e. ACCEPTANCE: neither depressed nor angry as these feelings have been expressed previously freeing the individual to deal with the handicap.

While the handicap of learning disabilities is usually not discerned until the school years, the lack of learning precipitates parents into anxieties, guilt, recriminations, and all the other feelings that occur when one is faced with the problems the child exhibits. The mourning process as described above lists the stages that parents live through as they attempt to uncover and remediate the difficulties that are arising in their child(ren).

Learning disabilities have a number of causes, etc. Some of the conditions that lead to learning difficulties can be inherited, as for example:

> Mrs. Z. contacted me because of concerns about her nine-year-old daughter Jane. Jane has a mild hearing loss in her left ear just as her mother. Both have had difficulty with mathematics as well as with developing friends. Both were described as immature and having difficulty understanding the social situation. The mother was seeking help for her daughter so that Jane would not have the same kind of unhappy childhood that Mrs. Z. had to weather. Mrs. Z. described the hearing/auditory problems as genetic, affecting only the females in her family.

Some of the conditions are acquired, that is the child has acquired the condition that no one else in the family has, for example:

> Fifteen-year-old Karen was born with a draining ear. As early as possible tubes were placed in her ears because of chronic, recurrent ear infections. However, her ears drained so much that the tubes soon plugged up and hence the chronic otitis media and the hearing loss persisted. She was diagnosed as learning disabled early in her school career with both auditory processing problems and a mild language disorder. No one else in her family has ear problems.

Other children develop learning disabilities as a result of closed head injuries. For example:

> As five-year-old Sally was being born, and her head had been partially delivered, the nurse held her back from coming completely through the birth canal. As a result of this action, Sally suffered rather diffuse damage to both hemispheres of her brain. She had a severe language handicap that was diagnosed as aphasia, did not understand that talking was for communication, and could not organize what she saw so that she could understand the world better.
>
> Sammy, four-years-old, suffered a closed head injury in a car accident when he was less than a year old, losing the sight in one eye as a result. According to his mother, Mrs. D., he lost all functions he had acquired. Sammy has had a great deal of rehabilitation from speech pathologists, physical therapists, and occupational therapists. While he is talking at this point he is not always understandable and there is still much jargon in his communications. He understands that talking is for communication and chatters away with others, expecting a response, often throwing a temper tantrum when he does not get the response he expects. However, his behavior is more like a two-and-a-half-year-old than a four-year-old.

As parents describe their children, they express a great deal of guilt and grief. Many of the mothers were the sole support of their handicapped child. They sought assistance and helped their child single-handedly. The fathers were seen as unwilling or unable to deal with the emotional toll of the reality of their child's condition. The mothers were still mourning the loss of their dreams for the child as well as dealing with their "if onlys." While consulted about the child, it is apparent that the parent is in need of help as well. There is a professional dilemma; what do you do first?

Since children grow in families and do best when both parents are involved in their rearing, it is important to reestablish the parental functions, and since it is Mother who has made contact, and since she is the one who is most overtly hurting, that is where to start. Drawing Father into the process is the next step even though Father seems to be handling himself adequately.

That he is divorced from the help/remediation seeking, suggests that his feelings may overwhelm him, which he handles by divorcing them as a means to function adequately on a day-to-day basis. While the child may need psychological help as do her/his parents, other remediation interventions can be instituted as parents are being helped to find their empathy for, and understanding of the child once again.

Helping Parents

A child does not stand alone. Rather, she/he is part of a constellation of interacting relationships known as a family. How a family functions is dependent upon how parents respond to the variety of characteristics their children exhibit. It is this responsiveness that can inhibit or enhance the social, emotional, and intellectual development of the child, handicapped or not. This means that the needs, feelings, and struggles of the parents must be handled, sometimes even before the rehabilitation of the child.

In our society, we are not educated to help the person who is grieving. The strong emotions that are expressed upon experiencing a loss embarrass us, make us feel helpless, and leave us feeling inadequate. These feelings more often than not lead us to withdraw from the grievers and encourage them to put these feelings aside and take up the routines necessary for living. However, people can only be in one place at a time. When they respond to your encouragement to put their grieving aside and continue their lives they can neither finish their grieving, nor become involved in the next step of living. They are in a kind of no-man's-land. As professionals, we need to help parents work through the grieving even though the expressions of grief lead us to feel helpless. That is part of the grieving process. Our feelings of helplessness are a reflection of the parents' feelings of helplessness. We can be with other people, we can walk with them on their trip through the grief, but we cannot do the work for them. Their task is to work through the grief, for without this process, old feelings and dreams cannot be put away so that the child that is can be responded to for her/himself. In other words attunement to the child and not the parental dream is crucial. The greatest help, therefore, is to listen and be there for the grieving person and not hurry them through their feelings.

Once some of the grieving has been accomplished, parents will be in a better position to become engaged in the rehabilitation process with the child and the variety of professionals being used to help the family. However, most professionals want to work with the child themselves. Helping a child grow and develop provide professionals a great deal of satisfaction that would be watered down were it to be shared with someone else. Parents, by virtue of their greater involvement with the child can enhance or sabotage the efforts of all professionals. Having parents as allies is our greatest help in the rehabilitation process. Using parents as cotherapists not only makes our jobs easier, but also enhances the process. This is a child-centered approach to the treatment/rehabilitation of the child. As professionals we can translate our understanding of the child into behavioral terms that we then share with the parents to help them develop more empathic bonds. Too often, we also have to do this same translating for other professionals to develop greater empathy for their young charges. In a report from a reading specialist and psychologist on a young child who was having difficulty learning to read it stated that the child exhibited inappropriate social behavior. The speech pathologist who was evaluating her noted that in the middle of testing the youngster would ignore her questions and make all kinds of social comments. This suggested to the examiner the child was having difficulty in understanding appropriate behavior as was stated in the report. When level of the test material became more difficult, the speech pathologist and the psychologist were able to discern that the child was beginning to fail. Reframing the child's behavior in light of the tasks she had to deal with as well as the comments by the mother that she did well socially and was well liked by her peers, the professionals were able to come up with an alternative explanation of the "inappropriate" behaviors. The youngster had success socially that she was affirming under conditions of failure. Rather than her behaviors being unsuitable for the situation, she was affirming that she was competent by demonstrating her ability to function well socially and distracting the examiner from asking the very questions she knew she would fail. She minimized her feelings of inadequacy by using her strengths. This behavior arose out of competence rather than inadequacy. The speech pathologist was very responsive to this reformulation and could see where other children who had exhibited similar kinds of maneuvers were making similar statements to her. She could then create other tactics to help children maintain positive self-images while helping them with their handicaps. The whole process that has just been described is one of the many ways in which parents and other professionals can be helped to develop a more empathic approach to children with whom they work.

Let us now look at the language-learning handicaps that have been discussed throughout this book.

Central Auditory Processing Disabilities (CAP)

Children with central auditory processing problems have learned not to listen because the auditory environment has been inconsistent for them. We are not talking about the normal four-year-old "deafness" where the child deliberately does not hear because what she/he is doing is far more important than what you want her/him to do. We are discussing children who do not know what sounds to respond to nor how to listen to sounds and words as was described in chapter 1 and 4.

The child with this disability is a challenge, not only for parents but for school personnel as well. What are the problems and how can they be dealt with? In chapter 4 we discussed the behavioral manifestations of this handicap; here we will discuss how those behaviors impact upon the people the child deals with on a day-to-day basis.

The child's inability to process/understand what she/he is hearing often generates many conflicts during the day. The parents feel that the child's "not listening" is deliberate. Responding to the behavior in anger, parents yell at the child, usually attacking her/him for incompetence and probably speaking at a faster pace than they usually speak. The child in turn gets angry, feels unloved and unappreciated, and incompetent (again). Once again she/he does not understand what the whole interchange was really about. This scenario repeated many times each day, every day has a deleterious impact upon the child and the family.

Unfortunately, we usually do not pick up central auditory processing problems until the child is beginning to have school difficulties especially with all aspects of the reading process: This occurs sometimes during first and second grade, but usually around fourth grade when children are expected to use higher-level processes of thinking. It is during this academic year that children are expected to begin to use more abstract levels of cognition and to generalize about their experiences and other forms of knowledge. Auditory-processing problems interfere with the maturation of this ability because the nature of this problem keeps children dependent upon the use of their vision to make sense of the world, just as it does the preconceptual child (see chapter 3). Let us go back to the Piagetian example of the tall skinny and short fat glass with the water being poured from one to another. The tall skinny glass really looks as if it had more water than the short fat glass. We know it is the same amount of water because we can explain to ourselves that no water was added or subtracted. The child, rooted in understanding the world visually, cannot explain this experiment in the way it has just been described. Rather she/he comes to the conclusion that the tall skinny glass has more water than the short fat glass. (Just think of how difficult it is to find an appropriate-sized container to hold the leftovers we wish to put away.) The inability to think through a problem keeps these children at the Piagetian preconceptual level of cognitive development. Since they cannot use language in the same way as their nonhandicapped peers they cannot automatically use their experiences and understandings for further growth. While these children need to be taught very specifically what nonhandicapped youngsters learn, seemingly by osmosis, too often we are unaware of the cognitive difficulty they are having. Rather, they present behavior problems at home, in school, and with peers that are seen as symptoms of "attention deficit disorders with hyperactivity" or as signs of emotional disturbance. From a psychological point of view, children with central auditory processing problems represent a class of children whose development has been arrested. This can be most patently seen in their friendship patterns. These children have difficult same-age relationships but get along with younger children with more comfort because they are functioning on approximately the same level. Unfortunately, the problematic behavior of these children often results in their being placed on medication to help them control these difficult behaviors. This course of action does not provide the child with the tools necessary to help them continue the very necessary emotional and cognitive growth. Psychotherapy can enable the child to begin to grow and develop emotionally. However, this child also needs help in learning how to think through an activity to which we often give little attention. While the psychotherapist can help the child grow emotionally and the school can help the child learn what is necessary to function in our society, it is the parents who must help the child learn how to listen and think. How can this be accomplished? Let's go back to the parents' frustration with their child's "not listening" mentioned above. The parents asked Johnny to go upstairs, wash his hands and face, change into his good clothes, and then come down again. A half hour later the child has still not reappeared so that one of the parents goes upstairs to find the child playing in his room, still unwashed and in his play clothes. Aggravating? Yes. How can this situation be handled so that the child can learn and grow from this experience without further damage to his already shaky self-esteem? First, the parent should find out what the child has heard and understood. More than likely the child has heard only the part about going upstairs. The parent should then explain that there were three other things that Johnny was asked to do and repeat them, giving reasons for the requests, e.g., we are going visiting or we are going to eat dinner in a restaurant, etc. Then the parent should tell Johnny what has to be done next. When the second request has been accomplished, the third, and then finally the last request, should be given. The parents need to understand that too many verbal requests overwhelm the child's processing abilities and hence one or maybe two will be remembered and the others forgotten. As the child handles one item consistently and accurately over a period of time a second activity can be added. The parents are training their child to listen. As explanations are given, they teach the child about cause-effect relationships, and about thinking. This provides the child with an empathic, supportive environment that not only supports her/his efforts and increases self-esteem but is respectful of the child.

Anger of the parents as a response to the child's behavior was mentioned earlier. In general it is a problematic feeling, but for the cap child it is disorganizing to her/his functioning. That is not to say that parents or any other people in interaction with the child should never get angry. The anger must be well controlled and well stated so that the expression and the handling of this difficult emotion can be understood by the child. When anger is expressed naturally with other children they usually understand what the feeling is and why the adults are angry. Not so the cap child. This child does not know whether to pay attention to the adult's behavior, the loudness of the voice or the words. The adult's controlled expression of feelings are designed to help the child understand and learn from the experience.

Whatever the situation, parents of CAP children need to explain carefully, slowly, and simply behaviors, feelings, cause-effect sequences, and outcomes to their children with as many visual clues and cues as is possible. In this way they are providing important learning/training in listening to the sequence of events in the environment, gaining information about what is happening, and enhancing self-esteem from being able to deal with the situation. In the long run they are learning how to learn.

Language Learning Disabilities

Language learning disabilities fall into three broad categories. The first that has been described above arises from central auditory processing problems. The second is usually, but not always, picked up early in the life of the child when her/his language production and understanding does not develop as expected. This child most frequently has difficulty learning how to read and write. The third arises out of a child's poor peer relationships and difficulty with arithmetic. We will be dealing with the language disordered child in this next section and the nonverbal (arithmetic) learning disordered child in the final section of this chapter.

When we think of language difficulties, problems in pronunciation or lack of speech usually come to mind. Some language disorders, however, can be very subtle and will also interfere with reading and other academic processes. For example:

> Tommy, nine years of age and in the fourth grade could barely read at a first-grade level. His teachers questioned his intellectual ability and referred him to the school psychologist for evaluation and possible placement in a mentally impaired classroom. His parents were angry with him because they thought he was willfully refusing to read. Behaviorally he got into a great deal of trouble and notes were continually sent home, even though they had no impact on the child's functioning. In desperation, the parents took him to a clinical child psychologist for a complete evaluation. The test findings indicated that the child, in addition to severe onslaughts against his self-esteem and sense of himself as a competent person, had a great deal of trouble handling verbal material. While he could eventually come up with the correct answer to questions he talked around the point until he could finally pinpoint what he wanted to say. At times he could not remember the word he wanted to use and needed help from the examiner to supply it for him. Based on these symptoms, the psychologist sent him for a complete speech, language, and neurological evaluation. The evaluation came back with some remarkable findings. This child had been living with a weakness on the right side of his body that had probably been there since birth. This finding suggested that Tommy had had a stroke, perinatally. The findings from the speech and language evaluation indicating a severe language disorder (aphasia) was consistent with the stroke. With this new information plans for the appropriate strategies to help Tommy learn more efficiently could be formulated.

Tommy's reading difficulties arose out of his basic language disability. In 1976 Vellutino[2] suggested that reading is a process dependent upon language, hence reading disabilities represent a variety of language disorders. At about the same time French, Rapin, et al.[3] in an attempt to disengage reading disabilities from minimal brain dysfunction did a massive study comparing brain-damaged individuals who had learned to read with brain damaged individuals who were unable to master this skill. They found three distinct groups:

1. Language disordered.
2. Language-motor disordered.
3. Visually disordered.

These findings digressed markedly from the then prevailing wisdom about reading-learning disabilities. However, in the ensuing years there has been a greater understanding that language problems of various forms are the underpinning for the reading disabilities we see.

Stevenson and Richman,[5] Baker and Cantwell,[6] and Love and Thompson[7] found a relationship between the presence of language delays and behavior problems beginning in the preschool years and lasting throughout the school years. According to a 1979 Carnegie Corporation[8] report, thought grows through language and conversely, language expresses thought. Without language concepts, generalization and abstractions cannot be developed. Peer relationships and shared play and fantasy do not occur. The child becomes a social isolate, and does not learn from peers what is appropriate behavior for her or his sex and age and develops more and more emotional difficulties. To illustrate:

> A mother was concerned about her three-and-one-half-year-old daughter who would not "mind." While discussing the problems Mrs. J. was having with her daughter, the youngster was playing with the dolls and dollhouse that was available for her. At a lull in the discussion with the mother the psychologist became aware that she could not understand the child's chattering. Mother remarked that the child always spoke that way and no one could understand her. The probability that the youngster's behavioral problems were related to the fact that the child was not talking at an age-appropriate level was noted and complete speech-language evaluation was recommended.
>
> Mary was six when her mother, given the diagnosis that her child was retarded, brain-damaged, and schizophrenic, followed through on a recommendation for psychotherapy. After seeing the child for once-a-week therapy, another psychologist was perplexed about the problems that the child was experiencing. She neither appeared retarded nor did she function as a schizophrenic child. In a parent conference, the mother mentioned that her older child was talking about getting a sundae from the ice cream parlor when Mary asked, "How could you get a 'sunday' when today is Tuesday?" Clearly, the child did not understand. The child was sent for a complete language evaluation, which concluded that she had a rather severe language disorder. This child was neither retarded nor schizophrenic.

> Nine-year-old Danny was referred for psychotherapy for rather explosive behavior that could not be contained. He was disrupting all the relationships within the family and creating a great deal of strain between his parents. His mother was quite protective of him and his father wanted to treat him with more severe limits than he currently had. When Danny did explode there was no way that an intervention by anyone in or out of the family could have an impact on him. During the course of treatment Mother was helped to be less protective of this child, and find an outlet professionally. Throughout the year and a half Danny was seen in treatment he matured and took greater responsibility for his own schoolwork although he still was not doing well. He continued to explode when he could not understand what was expected of him in classes requiring verbal skills. In discussions with his therapist it became increasingly apparent that Danny did not always understand what was said to him, or required of him. As his behavior came under better control he began to bite himself in frustration rather than explode. Therapy had helped him to institute better controls, feel that he was a worthwhile person, and gave him the inner strength to struggle through tasks that perplexed him most. Towards the end of treatment the psychologist decided that an evaluation of Danny's language abilities was in order. He was found to have a moderately severe word-finding difficulty that interfered with smooth and efficient academic functioning.

All of these children were labeled as emotionally disturbed because of behaviors that arose out of a variety of forms of language disorders. Remediating the language problem does not automatically clear up emotional difficulties that are expressed through the disordered behavior. Children with language problems, as well as children with central auditory processing problems, develop emotional disorders as the disordered language interferes with suitable cognitive and emotional growth.

The major emotional problem that parents need to be aware of and to deal with in the family is the language-disordered child's reliance on the parent to interpret the world to them, and them to the world. This reliance keeps the language disordered child more involved in intrafamilial relationships for longer periods of time than one would expect. The child's need to become increasingly autonomous is thwarted by her/his equally powerful need for the support and protection of the parents.

This chronic conflict that the child struggles with creates tensions and friction within the family. The empathic response needed by the child from the parents often gets eroded in the face of the continuing conflicts generated by the child's language disability. Both parents and child (and the other children in the family) should be in consultation with a clinical child psychologist or psychiatrist, who is familiar with the impact of language disorders on development to help them weather the inevitable emotional storms these children present. In the meantime, under some very adverse conditions, parents really need to keep their cool. As was mentioned above, while discussing central auditory processing problems a suggestion was made for parents to describe carefully, slowly, and in small doses, all the steps and stages necessary for the handicapped child to hear, understand, and process important material. This will begin to provide the child with skills to handle the environment and enhance her or his self-esteem. The same approach is necessary for the language-handicapped child, with modification. This child needs to have language used that is concrete and simple. Since these children are often very visually oriented, visual cues to supplement language may be necessary.

Some years ago at an interdisciplinary conference[9] devoted to children, a project was presented based on teaching young language-handicapped children how to sign. The researcher taught the children to use signs in addition to oral language in the same sequence that children learn how to use words (nouns, adjectives, verbs, etc.). They found that the children were able to express themselves better, lessening the incidence of emotional/behavioral problems. They were able to develop and maintain better relationships with parents, siblings, and other members of the family. They also developed and used language better than anyone expected. Signing words were not substituted for oral language, rather signing enhanced the children's language functions.

Nonverbal Learning Disabilities

A nonverbal learning disability, as described above, is usually brought to the attention of school personnel and parents when children are having trouble with peers. This usually occurs by the time the child is eight years old and in the third grade. Comments such as:

1. She/he doesn't know when to stop.
2. She/he's loud and bossy.
3. She/he interrupts, brags, and hogs the center of attention.
4. She/he blurts out inappropriate remarks.

By the time a child is eight she/he "should know better." As adults, we can say this to ourselves and be confident that we are correct. However, to say that to the child only shames her/him, creating anger and rage. This interferes with the child learning from the very person who wishes to help. Shaming them severs the relationship reducing the possibility of learning. It is only with relational bonds that children learn the important lessons and messages adults send to them. To return to the issue of "knowing better," when a child misbehaves or acts inappropriately, we as the adults must ask ourselves two questions:

1. What is going on in this situation that is causing the child to act in a disruptive manner?
2. Why isn't the child functioning better? This approach will give us far more information than thinking in terms of *shoulds* and *shouldn'ts*.

When one of the authors was about ten, she pointed some object out to her mother. Her mother's response to the query was, "Don't point with that finger." Needless to say, the ten year old was quite perplexed as she did not know which finger to use, nor was she given an alternative manner in which to designate the object she wanted to bring to her mother's attention. As adults we forget the perplexity we lived with as children when our own parents told us not to do something in a particular manner, yet expected us to behave differently. If we return to the child who has the symptoms described above we must give up the *shoulds* and look at the fact that the child has not been able to learn appropriate modes of functioning. The question now becomes, "Why is this so?"

There is a group of children who have a great deal of difficulty "reading" the social/interpersonal cues that most of us learn automatically. These children also have attendant problems dealing with arithmetic and mathematical skills and other understandings. According to Rourke[10] nonverbal learning disorders are evident by the time a child is eight or nine and are expressed in a variety of areas in addition to the difficulty "reading" social/interpersonal cues. These symptoms include:

a. Motor coordination difficulties.
b. Difficulties with visual-spatial-organizational abilities.
c. Deficits in nonverbal problem solving.
d. Difficulties in benefiting from either positive or negative feedback.
e. Difficulty with cause-effect relationships.
f. Does not/cannot respond to humor.
g. Does not adapt to new situations with ease, which leads to inappropriate behavior.
h. Significant difficulties with social perception, judgment, and interactional skills.
i. Social isolation with age.

These interpersonal/interactive problems leave these children vulnerable to the development of emotional difficulties. It therefore becomes necessary for environmental intervention to be instituted early. A prime intervention is the early identification of probable social/interaction difficulties. Since it is hard for parents to assess their own children's shortcomings, an outside observer needs to evaluate the child's interactions both with adults and peers. In addition to observation, the evaluator needs to look at the total context in which the child is functioning. In other words, the evaluator should look at whom the child is interacting with, what activity is the focus of the exchange, and then the sequence of events. This sequence of events is crucial as we can then begin to understand at which point the child's behavior "falls apart." When we have this data, then appropriate interventions can be developed to help the child learn more adequate and satisfying ways of interacting with others. We must remember that it is not a matter of the child knowing better, but that the child with a nonverbal learning disability has not been able to learn automatically about social interaction in the same way as children who do not suffer from nonverbal learning disorders.

The interventions developed to remediate the social problems these children exhibit need to include a strong experiential component. This would include role-playing interactions with an adult, at first to protect the child who has already been hurt by the rejections of peers. Videotaping of the role-play interaction would certainly add emphasis for the child as the adult and child discuss what happened in the interaction and the feelings that each person had during the exercise. As the child begins to comprehend the interactions with the adult, placing the child in a small group situation, again videotaped and reviewed after each interaction would be a good educational experience for all the children involved. Throughout the remediation process the child(ren) need help in learning how to put their feelings, thoughts, ideas into words rather than to express them overtly in behavior. At first, one would expect the nonverbal learning-disordered child to use the new learning in a stilted and possibly unthoughtful manner. These behaviors must also be corrected through direct experience as a way of helping the child learn how to function in a more appropriate and flexible social manner. In addition to new ways of interacting socially, this type of program must also help the child begin to think about her/his behavior in a more thoughtful manner. If new ways of thinking are not developed, the program has not been successful. Once the program is completed if the child does not have ways of thinking about new and novel situations she/he will not have skills to develop new approaches to new social encounters.

Since most children with this form of disability inevitably develop emotional problems, a thorough evaluation of emotional development is warranted. Recommendations for therapy may evolve from the assessment. The therapist chosen should be well aware of the nature of nonverbal learning disabilities and should be able to use role-playing with taping as one of her/his intervention strategies. In addition, the therapist should consider, at all times, the specific problems created by this disorder and use this knowledge in other interventions employed.

Parents must be an integral part of the entire intervention process. They aid in the process of helping the child return to the developmental track necessary for adequate growth in all areas of functioning.

Summary

Central auditory processing and language disorders impact on all areas of a child's life. Linguistic, social, and emotional development are dependent on a normal processing auditory system. Working as a team, the audiologist, speech-language pathologist, and clinical child psychologist cross fertilize their disciplines, and provide the disordered child with the most comprehensive and effective treatment available. The approach of the authors is based on developmentally expectable normal and age-appropriate linguistic, audiologic, cognitive, and emotional skills and behaviors.

An emphasis has been placed on appropriate and comprehensive evaluations by each of the disciplines represented here along with a complete medical assessment. Once data from all the evaluations are integrated remediation programs can be developed that are tailored to meet the specific needs of the child. Individually designed remediation programs must focus upon audiologic, linguistic, cognitive, and emotional factors both separately and integratively, as each area impacts upon the other. The ultimate goal of remediation is to enable the youngster to develop competency in all areas of functioning.

Given the research findings cited previously, that approximately 75 percent of children referred to mental health clinics for behavior problems suffer from some form of undiagnosed language/audiologic problems, one could assume that the ADHD diagnostic category should be placed under language disorders in the new *DSM-IV* manual, and should be treated as such. Just prescribing Ritalin or Cylert for the child is like putting calamine lotion on an itchy rash. Treating the symptom, not the underlying problem can only perpetuate the disorder rather than remediate the underlying problem. The child neither grows out of the problem with this form of topical medication nor does she/he grow out of the problem.

Language learning disabilities are lifelong and not confined to only kindergarten through twelfth grades. The world is full of learning disabled adults at all levels of functioning. How well a disabled adult performs depends upon the skills she/he has been able to develop and the degree of positive self-esteem the person feels.

Helping children become adults contributing to society depends upon appropriate and well-planned intervention programs instituted early in the academic careers of our children. A good remediation-intervention program that changes to match the growth and development of children with CAP and language disorders will enhance the skills and coping strategies so necessary to maneuver through the academic and social environments successfully.

This book has presented an interdisciplinary approach to the problems of language-learning disabilities and hyperactivity. For the authors, the interdisciplinary team includes teachers and parents as an integral part of the remediation process. Towards that end, this book has focused on "how to" and "what to do" by all parties interested in the best interests of the child after a thorough, professional assessment in all areas of functioning has been accomplished. Throughout the process, evaluation and remediation has been individualized to meet the specific needs of the specific child who must function within the environments of the family, the school, and with peers. Our recommendations have focused upon the enhancement of skills in each milieu that will lead to increased feelings of competence by the child, which can only enhance self-esteem.

Notes

Chapter 1: Auditory Development

1. F.H. Bess and A. Tharpe (1986) Case History Data on Unilaterally Hearing Impaired, *Ear and Hearing* 7 (1): pp. 14–7.

2. Jane Culbertson and L. Gilbert (1986) Children with Unilateral Sensori-Neural Hearing Loss: Cognitive, Academic and Social Development, *Ear and Hearing* 7 (1): pp. 38–51.

3. T.M. Klee and E. Davis-Dansky (1986) A Comparison of Unilaterally Hearing Impaired Children and Normal Hearing Children on a Battery of Standard Language Tests, *Ear and Hearing* 7 (1): pp. 27–37.

4. H. Needleman (1977) Effects of Hearing Loss From Early Recurrent Otitus Media on Speech and Language Development. In *Hearing Loss in Children,* B. F. Jaffe, ed. (Baltimore: University Park Press).

5. P. Menyuk (1980) Effect of Persistent Otitus Media on Language Development, *Anals of Otology, Rhinology, Larynology* 89: pp. 257–63.

6. P.W. Zinkus, M. Grottlieb and M. Shapiro (1978) Developmental and Psychoeducational Sequelae of Chronic Otitus Media, *American Journal of Disabilities in Children* (132) pp. 1100–4.

7. P.J. Brandes and D.M. Ehinger (1981) The Effects of Early Middle Ear Pathology on Auditory Perception and Academic Achievement, *Journal of Speech and Hearing Disorders* 43: pp. 301–7.

8. R.B. Eisenberg (1965) Auditory Behaviors in the Human Neonate I. Methodological Problems and the Logical Design of Research Procedures, *Journal of Audiological Research* 5: pp. 159–77.

9. R.B. Eisenberg (1969) Auditory Behavior in the Human Neonate. Functional Properties of Sound and Their Ontogenic Implications, *International Audiology* 9: pp. 34–45.

10. A Gesell and C. Armatruda (1947) *Developmental Diagnosis* (New York: Paul B. Hoeber, Inc).

11. E. Hardy (1965) Evaluation of Hearing in Infants and Young Children, in Glorig, A. *Audiometry, Principles and Practices* (Baltimore: Williams and Wilkins Co).

12. K. Murphy (1969) The Psychophysiological Maturation of Auditory Function. *International Audiology* 8: pp. 46–51.

13. J. Hardy, A. Dougherty and W. Hardy (1959) Hearing Responses and Audiologic Screening in Infants, *Journal of Pediatrics* (55) pp. 382–90.

14. E. Walden (1973) Audio-reflexometry in Testing of Very Young Children, *Audiology* (12) pp. 14–20.

15. R. Eisenberg (1970) The Organization of Auditory Behavior, *Journal of Speech and Hearing Research* (13) pp. 453–71.

16. B. Birns (1965) Individual Differences in Human Neonates' Responses to Stimulation, *Child Development* (36) pp. 249–56.

17. D. Ling (1972) Acoustic Stimulus Duration in Relation to Behavioral Responses of Newborn Infants, *Journal of Speech and Hearing Research* (15) pp. 567–71.

18. Pamela Gillet (1970) Auditory Processing, *Academic Therapy Publications* Novato, California.

19. American Psychiatric Association, *Diagnostic Statistical Manual*, 3rd edition (1987) Washington, DC.

20. Thomas Kenny (1989) A Tale of Two Systems: Children's Issues in England, A.P.A., *Division 37 Newsletter* 12 (4): 1989 pp. 1–4.

21. Alfel Kohn (1989) Suffer the Restless Children, *Atlantic Monthly* (Nov): pp. 90–100.

Chapter 2: Speech and Language Development

1. F. Williams, R. Hopper and D. Natalicio (1977) *Sounds of Children* (Harper & Row, New York) p. 2.

2. Eric Lenneberg (1966) The Natural History of Language. In F. Smith and P. Miller, eds., *The Genesis of Language* (Cambridge, Mass.: MIT Press) pp. 10–52.

3. R. Hopper and R. Naremore (1978) *Children's Speech: A Practical Introduction to Communication Development* 2nd ed. (New York, N.Y., Harper & Row, Inc) pp. 12–18.

4. J. Miller, R. Chapman, M. Branston and J. Ruchle (1980) Language Comprehension in Sensorimotor Stages 5 and 6, *Journal of Speech and Hearing Research* (4): pp. 11–20.

5. J. deVilliers and P. deVilliers (1979) *Early Language* (Cambridge: Harvard University Press) pp. 3–42.

6. Robert Owens (1984) *Language Development, an Introduction* (Columbus: Charles E. Merrill Publishing Co) pp. 19–36.

7. Lon Emerick and Charles VanRiper (1984) *Speech Correction: An Introduction to Speech Pathology and Audiology* (Englewood Cliffs, New Jersey: Prentice-Hall, Inc.) pp. 5–60.

8. P. Eimas (1974) Linguistic Processing of Speech by Young Infants. In R. Schiefebusch and L. Tenya, eds., *Language Perspectives—Acquisition, Retardation, and Interentions* (Baltimore: University Park Press) pp. 47–83.

9. Joseph Lichtenberg (1978) Psychoanalysis and Infant Research (New Jersey Analytic Press) pp. 126–73.

10. R. Hopper and R. Naremore (1978) *Children's Speech, a Practical Introduction to Communication Development* (New York: Harper & Row Publishers) pp. 23–33.

11. Barbara Wood (1976) *Children and Communication: Verbal and Nonverbal Language Development* (Englewood Cliffs, New Jersey: Prentice-Hall, Inc.) pp. 20–150.

12. Paula Meynuk (1971) *The Acquisition and Development of Language* (Englewood Cliffs: Prentice-Hall) pp. 78–9.

13. P. Dale (1976) *Language Development: Structure and Function* (New York: Holt, Rinehart and Winston) pp. 3–39.

14. C. Snow (1977) The Development of Conversation between Mothers and Babies, *Journal of Child Language* (4): pp. 1–22.

15. M. Braine (1976) Children's First Word Combinations, *Monographs of the Society for Research in Child Development* 41 pp. 11–31.

16. Roger Brown (1973) *A First Language: The Early Stages* (Cambridge: Harvard University Press) pp. 2–61.

17. Willard Quine (1964) Speaking of Objects. In J. Fordor and J. Katz, eds., *The Structure of Language* (Englewood Cliffs: Prentice-Hall) pp. 10–23.

18. D. Slobin (1973) Cognitive Prerequisites for the Development of

Grammar. In C. Ferguson and D. Slobin, eds. *Studies of Child Language Development* (New York: Holt, Rinehart & Winston) pp. 46–82.

19. E. Clark (1973) What's in a Word? On the Child's Acquisition of Semantics in His First Language. In T. Moore, ed. *Cognitive Development and Acquisition of Language* (New York: Academic Press) pp. 112–32.

20. M. Bowerman (1974) Discussion Summary, Development of Concepts Underlying Language. In R. Schiefebusch and L. Floyd, eds., *Language Perspectives—Acquisition, Retardation, and Intervention* (Baltimore University Park Press) pp. 120–42.

21. Dell Hymes (1972) Introduction in Courtney Cazden, Vera John, and Dell Hymes eds., *Functions of Language in the Classroom* (New York: Teachers College Press) p. 1.

22. J. Bruner (1975) The Ontogenesis of Speech Acts, *Journal of Child Language*, pp. 1–19.

23. R. Allen and K. Brown, eds. (1976) *Developing Communication Competence in Children* (Skokie, Illinois: National Textbook) pp. 15–36.

24. M. Haliday (1975) *Learning How to Mean: Explorations in the Development of Language* (New York: Edward Arnold) pp. 41–73.

25. C. Simon (1984) *Evolution of Language Competence* (Columbus, Ohio: Charles E. Merrill) pp. 27–83.

26. E. Wing and E. Semel *Language Assessment and Intervention for the Learning Disabled*, 2nd ed. (Columbus, Ohio: Charles E. Merrill) pp. 42–110.

27. David McNeil (1970) *The Study of Developmental Linguistics* (New York: Harper & Row) p. 21.

28. H. Francis (1972) Toward an Explanation of the Syntagmatic-paradigmatic Shift, *Child Development* (43): pp. 949–58.

29. J. Anglin (1970) *The Growth of Meaning* (Cambridge: MIT Press) pp. 16–40.

30. R. Owens (1984) *Language Development* (Columbus, Ohio: Charles E. Merrill Pub. Co.) pp. 230–97.

31. J. Piaget (1954) Language and Thought from the Genetic Point of View. *Acta Psychologica* (10): pp. 88–98.

32. B. White (1975) Critical Influences in the Origins of Competence *Merrill-Palmer and Warterly* (12): pp. 243–66.

33. T. Shultz (1974) Development of the Appreciation of Riddles, *Child Development* (45): pp. 100–5.

34. R. Lakoff (1973) Language, a Woman's Place, *Language of Sociology* (2): pp. 75–80.

35. M. Swacher (1975) The Sex of the Speaker as a Socialinguistic Variable. In B. Thorne and N. Henley, eds., *Language and Sex: Difference and Dominance* (Romley, Mass.: Newberry House: pp. 33–50.

36. M. Parlee (1979) Conversational Politics, *Psychology Today* (5): pp. 48–56.

37. L. Bloom (1975) Language Development. In F. Horowitz, ed., *Review of Child Development Research*, 4, (Chicago; Univeristy of Chicago Press) pp. 6–40.

38. E. Bates (1976) *Language and Context: The Acquisition of Pragmatics* (New York: Academic Press) pp. 47–131.

Chapter 3: Cognitive and Emotional Development of Children

1. Jean Piaget (1959) *Language and Thought in the Child* (New York: New World Publishing) pp. 1–288.

2. Richard M. Restak (1986) *The Infant Mind* (New York: Doubleday & Co., Inc.) pp. 1–274.

3. *Oxford English Dictionary* (1955) (London EC4: Oxford University Press).

4. T. Berry Brazelton (1981) *On Becoming Family* (New York: Delta/ Seymore Lawrence) pp. xi–210.

5. Nova Program-Life's First Feeling, "PBS."

6. J. Lichtenberg (1983) *Psychoanalysis and Infant Research* (New Jersey: Analytic Press) pp. 3–262.

7. Hildy S. Ross and Susan P. Laelis as reported in *Psychology Today* (October 1987): p. 14.

8. Thomas J. Freeburgand Marcia Z. Lippan (1986) Factors Affecting Discrimination of Infant Cries. *Journal of Child Language* (13) pp. 3–13.

9. Lynne Murray and Colwyn Trevarthen (1986) The Infant's Role in Mother-Infant Communications. *Journal of Child Language*, (13) pp. 15–29.

10. Lev Vygotsky (1986) *Thought and Language*, Alex Kozulin, trans. (Cambridge, London: MIT Press) pp. 1–168. Original work published 1934.

11. Lev Vygotsky (1978) *Mind in Society,* AR. Luria, trans. (Cambridge, London: Harvard University Press) pp. 1–159.

12. A. R. Luria and F. I. Yudovich (1966) *Speech and Development of Mental Processes in the Child,* O. Kovasc and J. Simon, trans. (London: Staples Press) pp. 20–110. (Original work published 1956).

13. Norbert Freedman (1977) Hands, Words and Mind: On the Structuralization of Body Movements during Discourse and the Capacity for Verbal Representation. In Norbert Freedman and Standley Grand, eds., *Communicative Structures and Psychic Structures* (New York and London: Plenum Press) pp. 109–32.

14. J. Brunere (1966) *Towards a Theory of Instruction* (Cambridge-Belknap Press) pp. 1–176.

15. P. Lindsay and D. Norman (1977) *Human Information Processing,* 2nd ed. (New York: Academic Press) pp. 1–712.

16. Burton White (1985) *The First Three Years of Life,* (New York: Prentice Hall Press) pp. 1–285.

17. Samuel Karelitz and Vincent R. Fisichelli (1962) The Cry Thresholds of Normal Infants and Those with Brain Damage, *Journal of Pediatrics* 61 (5): pp. 679–85.

18. Vincent R. Fisichelli and Samuel Karelitz (1963) The Cry Latencies of Normal Infants and Those with Brain Damage, *Journal of Pediatrics* 62 (5): pp. 724–34.

19. E. Erikson (1950) *Childhood and Society* (New York: W. W. Norton & Co.) pp. 7–445.

20. Robert White (1959) Motivation reconsidered: The Concept of Competence, *Psych. Rev.* 66: pp. 297–333.

21. Katrina de Hirsch (1975) Language Deficits in Children with Developmental Lags. In Ruth S. Eissler, Anna Freud, Marianne Kris, Albert J. Solnit, eds. *The Psychoanalytic Study of the Child,* 30, pp. 95–126 (New Haven: Yale University Press).

22. E. Buchholz (1989) The Legacy from Childhood: Considerations for Treatment of the Adult with Learning Disabilities, *Psychoanalytic Inquiry,* pp. 431–52.

23. S. Fraiberg (1959) *The Magic Years* (New York: Chas Anderson & Sons) pp. 3–305.

24. G. H. Bachara and J. N. Zaba (1975) Learning Disabilities and Juvenile Delinquency *Journal of Learning Disabilities* 11: pp. 242–46.

25. B. A. Lane (1980) The Relationship of Learning Disabilities to Juvenile Delinquency: Current Status *Journal of Learning Disabilities* 13 pp. 425–34.

26. *Carnegie Quarterly* (1979) 27 (1) Winter: pp. 1–12.

Chapter 4: Language Learning Disabilities Identification and Evaluation

1. R. J. Ruben (1979) Introduction: Workshop in Otitus Media and Development, *Annals of Otology, Rhinology, Laryngology*, pp. 3–12.

2. L. Fisch (1983) Integrated Development and Maturation of the Hearing System. A critical review article, *British Journal of Audiology* 17: pp. 137–54.

3. D. Webster and M. Webster (1977) Neonatal Sound Deprivation Affects Brainstem Auditory Nuclei, Arch. Otolaryngol, 103.

4. R. A. Dobie and C. I. Berlin (1979) Influence of Otitus Media on Hearing and Development, *Ann. Otol. Rhinol. Laryngol*, 88: pp. 48–53, suppl. 60.

5. W. T. Greenough (1975): Experiential Modification of the Developing Brain, *Am. Sci.* 63: pp. 37–46.

6. V. A. Holm and L. H. Kunze (1969) Effects of Chronic Otitus Media on Language and Speech Development, *Pediatrics*, 43: pp. 833–39.

7. G. K. Kaplan, J. K. Fleshman, T. R. Bender et al. (1973) Long-term Effects of Otitus Media: A Ten Year Cohort Study of Alaska Eskimo Children, *Pediatrics* 52: pp. 577–85.

8. D. Lewis (1976) Otitus Media and Linguistic Incompetence, *Archives of Otolaryngology* 102: pp. 387–90.

9. H. Needleman (1977) Effects of Hearing Loss from Early Recurrent Otitus Media on Speech and Language Development. In *Hearing Loss in Children*,B. J. Jaffee, ed. (Baltimore: University Park Press).

10. P. Menyuk (1980) Effects of Persistent Otitus Media on Language Development, *Annals of Otology, Rhinology, Laryngology* 89: pp. 257–63.

11. P. Zinkus, M. Gottlieb and M. Shapiro (1978) Developmental and Psychoeducational Sequelae of Chronic Otitus Media, *American Jour. of Disabilities in Children* 132: pp. 1100–4.

12. P. Brandes and D. Ehinger (1981) The Effects of Early Middle Ear Pathology on Auditory Perception and Academic Achievement, *Journal of Speech and Hearing Disorders*, pp. 301–4.

13. L. Masters and G. Marsh (1978) Middle Ear Pathology as a Factor in Learning Disabilities, *Journal of Learning Disabilities* 11: pp. 54–7.

14. F. C. Bennett, S. H. Ruuska and R. Sherman (1980) Middle Ear Function in Learning Disabled Children, *Pediatrics* 66 2: pp. 254–60.

15. Mary Ellen Brandell and Linda Seestedt (1979) Hearing Loss and Its Effect on Language Learning. (Research Paper)

16. E. Bocca, C. Calearo and V. Cassinari (1954) A New Method for Testing Hearing in Temporal Lobe Tumors, *Acta. Orolaryngol* 44: pp. 219–21.

17. J. Jerger (1960) Audiological Manifestations of Lesions in the Auditory Nervous System, *Laryngoscope* 70: pp. 417–25.

18. J. Katz (1962) The Use of Staggered Spondaic Words for Assessing the Integrity of the Central Auditory Nervous System, *Journal of Auditory Research* 2: pp. 327–37.

19. J. Willeford (1978) Sentence Tests of Central Auditory Function. In J. Katz, ed. *Handbook of Clinical Audiology*, 2nd ed. (Baltimore: Williams & Wilkins) pp. 252–61.

20. Robert Keith (1986) SCAN: A Screening Test for Auditory Processing Disorders (The Psychological Corp. Harcourt Brace Jovanovich) 1986.

21. M. A. K. Halliday (1975) Training How to Fear: Explorations in the Development of Language (Edward Arnold Put. Ltd.) pp. 26–53.

22. M. A. K. Halliday (1978) Language as Social Semiotic (Baltimore: University Park Press) pp. 3–26.

23. B. Berereiter and S. Engelmann (1966) *Teaching Disadvantaged Children in the Preschool* (Englewood Cliffs, New Jersey: Prentice-Hall) pp. 18–69.

24. J. Piaget (1955) *The Language and Thought of the Child*, translated by M. Sabian (Cleveland: Meredian Press) pp. 1–52.

25. I. Z. Sigel and R. R. Cosking, (1977) *Cognitive Development from Childhood to Adolescence* (New York: Holt, Rinehart and Winston) pp. 1–76.

26. E. Wiig and E. M. Semel, (1976) *Language Disabilities in Children*

and Adolescents (Columbus, Ohio: Charles E. Merrill Publ. Co.) pp. 42–131.

27. E. Wiig and E. M. Semel, (1980) *Language Assessment and Intervention for the Learning Disabled* (Columbus, Ohio: Charles E. Merrill) pp. 16–173.

28. C. Simon (1985) *Communicative Skills and Classroom Success: The Language Learning Disabled Student: Description and Therapy Implications* (San Diego: College Hill Press) pp. 1–56.

29. N. S. Rees (1978) *Pragmatics of Language in Bases of Language Intervention*, R. L. Shelferbusch, ed. (Baltimore: University Park Press) pp. 73–112.

30. N. Speckman and F. Roth (1984) Clinical Evaluation of Language Functions (CELF) Diagnostic Battery: An Analysis and Critique, *Journal of Speech and Hearing Disorders* 49: pp. 94–111.

31. R. Lieberman and A. Michael (1986) Content Relevance and Content Coverage in Tests of Grammatical Ability, *Journal of Speech and Hearing Disorders* 51: pp. 71–81.

32. American Speech Language and Hearing Association 1989 ASHA.

33. P. Broen and G. Siegel (1976) "Language Assessment" in Communication, *Assessemtn and Intervention Strategies*, L. L. Loyd, ed. (Baltimore: University Park Press) pp. 76–109.

34. N. Rees and M. Shulman (1978) I Don't Understand What You Mean by Comprehension, *Journal of Speech and Hearing Disorders* 43 2: pp. 202–19.

35. J. M. Gallagher and I. J. Quandt (1981) Piaget's Theory of Cognitive Development and Reading Comprehension: A New Look at Questioning, *Topics in Learning and Learning Disabilities*, 1 (1): pp. 21–30.

36. S. Ervin-Tripp (1977) Wait for Me, Roller-Skate. In S. Ervin-Tripp and C. Mitchell-Kernan, eds. *Child Discourse* (New York: Academic Press) pp. 23–62.

37. N. Lupert (1981) Auditory Perceptual Impairments in Children with Specific Language Disorders. A Review of the Literature, *Journal of Speech and Hearing Research* 46 (1): pp. 3–9.

38. M. D. Berry and R. L. Erickson (1973) Speaking Rote: Effects on Children's Comprehension of Normal Speech, *Journal of Speech and Hearing Research* 16 (3): pp. 367–74.

39. E. Z. Lasky and A. M. Chapandy (1976) Factors Affecting Language Comprehension, *Language, Speech, and Hearing Services in the Schools* 7 (3): pp. 159–68.

40. Charlarn Simon (1986) Evaluating Communicative Competence (Communication Skills Builders, Inc.) pp. 3–149.

41. J. Tough (1979) *Listening to Children Talking* (London: Ward Loch Educational) pp. 16–52.

42. R. E. Bassett, N. Whittington and A. Staton-Spicer (1978) The Basics in Speaking and Listening for High School Graduates: What Should Be Assessed? *Journal of Communication Disorders* 27: pp. 298–302.

43. W. Loban (1976) Language Development: K-12 (Urbana, Illinois: National Council of Teachers of English) pp. 5–12.

44. J. Flood and M. W. Salus (1982) Metalinguistic Awareness: Its Role in Language Development and Assessment, *Topic in Language Disorders* 2 (4): pp. 56–64.

45. J. R. Johnston (1982), Narratives: A New Look at Communication Problems in Older Language Disordered Children, *Language, Speech, and Hearing Services in the Schools* 13(3): pp. 144–45.

46. C. Westby (1984) Development Narrative Language Abilities. In G. P. Wallace and K. S. Butler, eds., *Language Learning Disabilities in School Age Children* (Baltimore: Williams and Wilkins) pp. 87–123.

47. Arnold J. Love and Michael Thompson, G. G. (1988) Language Disorders and Attention Deficit Disorders in Young Children Referred for Psychiatric Services: Analysis of Prevalence and a Conceptual Synthesis, *Amer. J. Orthopsychiat.* 58 (D), pp. 52–64.

48. G. H. Bachara and J. N. Zaba (1975) Learning Disabilities and Juvenile Delinquency, *J. of Learning Disabilities* 11: pp. 242–46.

49. B. A. Lane (1980) The Relationship of Learning Disabilities to Juvenile Delinquency: Current Status, *Journal of Learning Disabilities* 13: pp. 425–34.

Chapter 5: Treatment and Intervention

1. J. Sanders (1965) Noise Conditions in Normal School Classrooms, *Except. Child* 31: pp. 344–53.

2. R. L. Paul (1967) An Investigation of the Effectiveness of Hear-

ing Aid Amplification in Regular and Special Classrooms under Instructional Conditions (doctoral dissertation, Wayne State University).

3. R. Gengel (1971) Acceptable Speech to Noise-ratios for Aided Speech Discrimination by the Hearing Impaired, *J. Audit. Res.* 11: pp. 219–22.

4. T. Finitzo-Hiebert and T. Tillman (1978) Room Acoustics Effects on Monosyllabic Word Discrimination Ability for Normal and Hearing Impaired Children, *J. Speech Hearing Research* 21: pp. 440–58.

5. M. Ross (1972) Classroom Accoustics and Speech Intelligibility. In J. Katz, ed., *Handbook of Clinical Audiology* (Baltimore: Williams & Wilkins) pp. 756–71.

6. R. Blake; C. Torpey and P. Wertz (1987) *Effects of FM Auditory Trainers in Attending Behaviors of Learning Disabled Children, Preliminary Findings* (Telex Communications).

7. L. Sarff (1981) An Innovative Use of Free Field Amplification in Regular Classrooms. In *Auditory Disorders in School Children*, ed. Roesner and Downs, (New York: Theime-Stratton, Inc.).

8. D. Gibson and D. Ingram (1983) The Onset of Comprehension and Production in a Language Delayed Child, *Applied Psycholinguistics* 4: pp. 359–76.

9. L. Olswang and T. Coggins (1986) The Effects of Adult Behaviors on Increasing Language Delayed Children's Production of Early Relationship Meanings, *British Journal of Disorder of Communication* 19: pp. 18–34.

10. Olswang, et al. (1986) Language Learning: Moving Performance from a Context-dependent to Independent State, *Child Language Teaching and Therapy* 2: pp. 180–210.

11. P. Menyuk (1975) Children with Language Problems: What's the Problem? In *Developmental Psycholinguistics: Theory and Applications* (Washington: Georgetown University Press) pp. 129–44.

12. P. Tallal (1988) *Developmental Language Disorders in Learning Disabilities: Proceedings of the National Converence* eds., J. Kavanagh and T. Truss, (Parkton, Maryland: York Press).

13. M. Fey (1986) *Language Intervention with Young Children* (San Diego: College Hill Press) pp. 7–33.

14. M. Marge (1972) The Problem of Management and Corrective

Education. In *Principles of Childhood Language Disabilities* (New York: Appleton Century-Crafts) pp. 197–363.

15. L. McCormick and R. Goldman (1984) Designing an Optimal Learning Program. In L. McCormick and R. Schiefebusch, eds., *Early Language Intervention* (Columbus: Charles E. Merrill Pub. Co.) pp. 202–41.

16. L. Leonard (1983) Defining the Boundaries of Language Disorders in Children. In J. Miller, D. Yoder and R. Schiefdeausch, eds., *Contemporary Issues in Language Intervention* (Rockville, Maryland: The Am. Speech and Hearing Association) pp. 107–12.

17. S. Warren and A. Kaiser (1986) Generalization of Treatment Efforts by Young Language Disordered Children: A Longitudinal Analysis, *Journal of Speech and Hearing Disorders* 51: pp. 239–51.

18. Guess, et al. (1978) Children with Limited Language. In R. Schieflebusch, ed., *Language Intervention Strategies* (Baltimore: University Park Press.) pp. 101–43.

19. L. Vygotsky (1978) *Find in Society: The Development of Higher Psychological Processes* (Cambridge: Harvard University Press) pp. 26–37.

20. G. Gottlieb (1976) The Roles of Experience in the Development of Behavior and the Nervous System. In G. Gottlieb, eds., *Studies in the Development of Behavior and the Nervous System* (New York: Academic Press) pp. 25–54.

21. C. Wilson, Lanza, Jr. and J. Barton (1988) Developing Higher Level Thinking Skills Through Questioning Techniques in the Speech and Language Setting, *Language Speech and Hearing Services in the Schools* 19: pp. 428–31.

22. B. Bloom ed. (1956) *Taxonomy of Educational Objectives Handbook One: Cognitive Domain* (New York: McKay) pp. 23–114.

23. E. Wiig and E. Semel, *Language Disabilities in Children* pp. 1–132.

24. E. Wiig and E. Semel, *Language Assessment and Intervention* pp. 41–116.

25. M. Donahue and T. Bryon (1984) Communication Skills and Peer Relations of Learning Disabled Adolescents, *Topics in Language Disorders* 4: pp. 10–21.

26. J. Searle (1965) What is a Speech Act? In *Philosophy in American*, ed. M. Black (Ithaca, New York: Cornell University Press) pp. 34–51.

27. H. P. Grice (1975) *Logic and Conversation in Syntax and Semantics*, 3, *Speech Acts* ed., P. Cole and J. L. Morgan (New York: Academic Press) pp. 16–57.

28. R. Bourgault (1985) Mass media and Pragmatics: An Approach for Developing Testing, Speaking, Writing in Secondary Schools. In Simon, ed., *Conversation* (Skill College Hill Press) pp. 241–55.

29. C. Simon (1981) Communicative Competence: A Functional pragmatic Approach to Language, *Therapy Lesson* (Arizona: Communication Skill Builders) pp. 4–56.

30. C. Simon (1979) Philosophy for Learning Disabled Students, *Thinking: A Journal of Child Philosophy* l: pp. 21–34.

31. E. I. Hammer-Eden (1969) A Comparison of the Oral Language Patterns of Mature and Immature First Grade Children. (doctoral dissertation, Arizona State University, Tempe, Arizona).

32. D. R. Moore (1971) Language Research and Preschool Language Training. In *Language Training in Early Childhood Education*, C. S. Lantelli, ed. (Urbane, Illinois: University of Illinois Press) pp. 3–47.

33. C. O'Brien (1973) *The Language Different Child* (Columbus, Ohio: Charles C. Merrill) pp. 83–106.

34. M. Halliday (1978) *Language as Social Semiotic* (Baltimore: Unviersity Park Press) pp. 2–38.

35. R. VanAllen and C. VanAllen (1970) *An Introduction to Language Experiences in Language Land One*, Teacher Resource Book, (Encyclopaedia: Britannica Press) p. 5.

36. C. O'Brien (1985) First Steps in Reading for the Language Different Child. In C. Simon, eds., *Communication Skill and Classroom Success* (San Diego) pp. 273–94.

37. W. Shuy (1972) Speech Differences and Teaching Strategies: How Different Is Enough? In E. Hodges and E. H. Rudolph, eds., *Language and Learning to Read* (Boston—Houghton Mifflin) p. 281.

38. M. Zintz (1970) *The Reading Process: The Teacher and the Learner* (Dubuque, Iowa: William C. Brown Co.) pp. 1–210.

39. L. Olquin (1972) *Shuck Loves Chirley* (Pasadena, California: Original American Press) pp. 1–52.

40. Elaine A. Lasky (1985) *Comprehending and Processing Information in Clinic and Classroom in Communication Skills and Classroom Success*, ed.

Charlann Simon (San Diego, California: College Hill Press) pp. 281–312.

41. M. Blank (1974) Cognitive Functions of Language in the Preschool Years. *Developmental Psychology* 10: pp. 229–45.

42. A. R. Luria (1961) *The Role of Speech in the Regulation of Normal and Abnormal Behavior* (New York: Linerscript) pp. 12–22.

43. D. Danserean (1978) The Development of a Learning Strategies Curriculum. In H. F. O'Neil, ed., *Learning Strategies* (New York: Academic Press) pp. 126–67.

44. Ph.D. Lindsey and D. A. Norman (1972) *Human Informal Processing: An Introduction to Psychology* (New York: Academic Press).

45. B. J. Meyer (1975) *The Organization of Prose and Its Effects on Memory* (Amsterdam: North-Holland Publishing Co.).

46. J. Lichtenberg (1989) *Psychoanalysis and Motivation* (Hillsdale, New Jersey: The Analytic Press).

47. Brian Sutton-Smith (1971) *The Study of Games* (New York: John Wiley and Sons).

48. Reuven Feuerstein (1980) *Instrumental Enrichment* (Glenview, Illinois: Scott Foresman and Co.).

49. Nicholas Hobbes (1980) Feuerstein's Instrumental Enrichment; Teaching Intelligence to Adolescents, *Educational Leadership*, pp. 566–71.

Chapter 6: Families

1. Elisabeth Kübler-Ross (1976) *On Death and Dying* (New York: Macmillan Publishing Co) pp. 1–289.

2. Frank R. Vellutino (1979) *Dyslexia: Theory and Research* (London: MIT Press) pp. 1–427.

3. S. Mattis, J. French and I. Rapin (1975) Dyslexia in Children and Young Adults: Independent Neuropsychological Syndromes, *Developmental Medicine and Child Neurology*, 17 (2): pp. 150–63.

4. Selma Fraiberg (1959) *The Magic Years* (New York: Charles Scribner and Sons) pp. 3–305.

5. Jim Stevenson and Naomi Richman (1978) Behavior, Language,

and Development in Three Year Old Children, *J. of Autisum and Childhood Schizophrenia* 8 (3): pp. 299–304.

6. L. Baker and D. Cantwell (1982) Developmental, Social, and Behavioral Characteristics of Speech and Language Disordered Children, *Child Psychiatry and Human Development*, 12 (4): pp. 195–206.

7. Arnold S. Love and Michael G. Thompson (1988) Language Disorders and Attention Deficit Disorders in Young Children Referred for Psychiatric Services, *Amer. J. Orthopsychiatry* 58 (1): pp. 52–64.

8. Carnegie Corporation (1979) 27 (1): pp. 1–12.

9. American Association of Psychiatric Services for Children (1976) New Orleans.

10. Byron P. Rourke (1987) Syndrome of Nonverbal Learning Disabilities: The Final Common Pathway of White Matter Disease/Dysfunction, *Clinical Neuropsychologist* 1 (3): pp. 209–34.

Appendix A
Parent Suggestions

General Suggestions for Parents of Children with Central Auditory Processing Difficulties

1. Set aside specific times during the day to work with your child. Let these times be for you and your child alone.
2. Start with short work periods and gradually increase them. A good rule is to stop when your child is at the peak of success. Do not push the child to the point of failure.
3. Be as objective and patient as you can. Speak to your child in a quiet, firm voice.
4. Make commands or directions short and simple.
5. If a task is too difficult for your child, move on to something easier. Then come back to the first task after changing it so that your child can succeed.
6. When your child is capable of doing a task, gently insist that she/he finish it.
7. Be aware of your child's abilities as well as her/his weaknesses. Do not continue using tasks that are too easy for your child. There should be some challenge to hold your child's attention.
8. Praise your child for even the smallest success. Do not emphasize failures.
9. Really listen to your child. Be there when she/he needs your help.
10. Relax with your child. Enjoy your time together.
11. Be honest with your child. Do not say there is nothing wrong. No one knows better than your child that something is wrong with the way she/he learns.
12. Take a positive approach: "There is help. You can learn. Learning might seem slow for a while, but I am in this with you."
13. The last and most important tip is this: Be easy on yourself. You did not create your child's language learning disabilities. You can not handle everything at once. You are human. Sometimes you won't have the patience to work with your child. Sometimes you will feel like giving up. Don't. Ask for help when you need it.

Specific Suggestions

1. Structure the environment
   a. Attempt to foster cooperative and understanding relationships in the home. The child needs a stable base.
   b. Provide day-to-day, pleasant learning experiences of a formal or informal nature.
   c. Provide a calm, simple, austere decor.
   d. Use few mirrors and stimulating objects.
   e. Have the child's workplace facing a blank wall.
   f. Give every child a quiet corner of her/his own.
   g. Have a clear routine for the child. Construct a timetable for waking, eating, play, TV, study, chores, and bedtime. Follow it flexibly although she/he disrupts it. The structure will eventually reap benefits.
   h. Give your child responsibility, which is essential for growth. You may need to supervise her/him carefully. Acceptance and recognition of her/his efforts, even if imperfect, should not be overlooked.

2. Punishment
   a. Set consistent limits and standards.
   b. Do not punish a child for behavior that she/he cannot control, like clumsiness or frustration. Spankings are not recommended, for they teach a child not to misbehave in the adult's presence. It does not help her/him learn self-control.
   c. Punishment should be prompt and appropriate to the misbehavior.
   d. Avoid long discussions and logical reasoning. Handle the problem directly and simply.
   e. Do not spend excessive time punishing bad behavior at the expense of encouraging good behavior.
   f. Use a child's bed as a place of rest, not as a punishment site.
   g. If you wish to teach a child to hold his temper, then be able to exhibit that behavior yourself.
   h. Separate behavior that you do not like from the child's *person* that you do like. "I like you. I don't like your tracking mud through the house."
   i. Avoid a constant negative approach: "Stop" "Don't" "No." When saying no to something provide child with a more appropriate way of expressing her-/himself.
   j. Try to keep your emotions cool by preparing yourself for expectable turmoil. Recognize and respond to any positive behavior, however small. Search for good things; you'll find a few.

k. Use a quiet, low voice. Anger is normal and can be controlled. Anger does not mean you do not love the child.

3. Trouble Prevention
   a. Remove and prevent intolerable stimulation.
   b. Give simple, clear instructions in short series.
   c. When the child exhibits impatience about impending activities, help her/him by building a step-by-step inner picture. Describe in detail any and all facets of the activity, such as its purpose, any stops, and interesting sights to be expected.
   d. Anxious children can be made more comfortable about expected events if they are predictable as to time, place, etc. Meals should be at regular times, and activities can be scheduled somewhat consistently.
   e. Rules of behavior should be definite, simple and unchanging from parent to parent and time to time.
   f. Gradual increases in independence can be achieved by:
      1. Simple, useful needed household chores.
      2. Encouragement of special talents and interests.
   g. Demonstrate difficult tasks, using action accompanied by short, clear, quiet, explanations. Repeat the demonstration until the task is learned. Be patient.
   h. Establish, if possible, a separate room or part of a room that is the child's own, special area. Avoid brilliant patterns or complex patterns in decor. Keep clutter to a minimum.
   i. Do one thing at a time; give her/him one toy from a closed box. Clear the table of everything else when coloring. Turn off the radio/TV when the child is doing homework.
   j. Learn to read the child's explosive warning signals and intervene quietly to avoid these by distracting him or discussing the conflict calmly.
   k. Restrict playmates to one or two at most, at any one time. Your home is a more suitable play area because you can provide the structure and supervision needed. Explain your rules to the playmate(s) and briefly tell the other parent your reasons.
   l. Talk with your child about the meanings of jokes and riddles.
   m. Read a story with your child everyday. Ask questions about the story, letting your child tell you about his or her favorite part, the funniest part, the scariest part, and so on.

Appendix B
School Suggestions

Management/Treatment Strategies for the Child with Central Auditory Processing Difficulties

Children with auditory processing deficits typically demonstrate one or more of the following problems:

Poor auditory attending skills.

Deficits in foreground/background discrimination.

Limitations in auditory memory and retrieval.

Delays in receptive auditory language development.

These guidelines are based on strategies designed to minimize the impact of such problems upon academic achievement.

1. *Classroom Placement.* Determine the available options for classroom placement. Consider such critical factors as: the acoustics of the classroom relative to noise level and reverberation; the amount of structure within the classroom, and teacher's communication style. In general, a self-contained structured situation is more effective for children with auditory deficits than an open, unstructured teaching environment.

2. *Look and Listen.* Children with even mild auditory problems function much better in the classroom if they can both look and listen.

3. *Classroom Seating.* Preferential seating is a major consideration in managing such children. Children with auditory deficits should be assigned seats away from halls or street noise and not more than ten feet from the teacher. Such seating allows the child to better utilize hearing and visual cues. Flexibility in seating better enables the child to attend and actively participate in class activities.

In some cases, central auditory testing by the audiologist will reveal a significant difference in processing skills between the child's two ears. In such an instance preferential classroom seating so the child can favor the better ear is recommended.

Some audiologists also will recommend plugging the poorer ear with a custom-made earplug or earmuff as a means for improving the child's auditory function. At present there is no significant research either to support or refute this practice.

4. *Gain Attention.* Always gain the child's attention before giving directions or initiating class instruction. Calling the child by name or gently touching him/her will serve to alert the child and to focus attention upon the classroom activity.

5. *Check Comprehension.* Ask children with an auditory deficit questions related to the subject under discussion to make certain that they are following and understanding the discussion.

6. *Rephrase and Restate.* Encourage children with auditory-processing problems to indicate when they do not understand what has been said. Rephrase the question or statement since certain words contain sounds or blends that are not easily discriminated. Also, most children with auditory problems have some delay in language development and may not be familiar with key words. By substituting words and simplifying the grammar you may more readily convey the intended meaning.

7. *Use Brief Instructions.* Keep instructions relatively short; otherwise the child with a limited auditory memory span will be lost.

8. *Pretutor Child.* Have children read ahead on a subject to be discussed in class so that they are familiar with new vocabulary and concepts, and thus can more easily follow and participate in classroom discussion. Such pretutoring is an important activity that the parents can undertake.

9. *List Key Vocabulary.* Before discussing new material, list key vocabulary on the blackboard. Then try to build the discussion around this key vocabulary.

10. *Visual Aids.* Visual aids help children with limited auditory skills by capitalizing upon strengths in visual processing and thus providing the auditory visual association often necessary for learning new concepts and language.

11. *Individual Help.* Whenever possible, provide individual help in order to fill gaps in language and understanding stemming from the child's auditory problems.

12. *Quiet Study Areas.* Provide an individual study area relatively free from auditory and visual distractions. Such an area helps minimize the child's problem in foreground/background discrimination.

13. *Involve Resource Personnel.* Inform resource personnel of planned vocabulary and language topics to be covered in the classroom so that pretutoring can supplement classroom activities during individual therapy.

14. *Write Instructions.* Children with auditory problems may not follow verbal instructions accurately. Help them by writing assignments on the board so they can copy them in a notebook. Also, use a "buddy system" by giving a classmate the responsibility for making certain the child is aware of the assignments made during the day.

15. *Encourage Participation.* Encourage participation in expressive language activities such as reading, conversation, story telling, and creative dramatics. Reading is especially important, since information and knowledge gained through reading help compensate for what may be missed because of auditory deficits. Again, parents can assist the child through their participation in local library reading programs and carryover activities in the home.

16. *Monitor Efforts.* Remember that children with impaired auditory function become fatigued more readily than other children. Subsequently, they do not attend because of the continuous strain resulting from efforts to keep up and to compete in classroom activities. Therefore, provide short intensive periods of instruction with breaks during which the child can move around.

17. *Inform Parents.* Provide the parents with consistent input so that they understand the child's successes and difficulties, as well as the need for individual tutoring at home.

18. *Evaluate Progress.* Do not assume a program is working. Instead, evaluate the child's progress on a systematic schedule. It is far better to modify a program than to wait until a child has encountered yet another failure.

Glossary

Accommodation — Alteration of existing concepts to allow for the addition of new material.

Air Conduction — Measurement made with earphones of an audiometer that evaluates the entire hearing mechanism.

Articulation — Process for speech production that includes synchronized oral motor movements that result in vibration of the vocal folds.

Assimilation — New material is added onto already established concepts without modification of the concept.

Audiogram — A graph depicting the level of hearing an individual has for particular tones. An audiogram is done to assess a person's peripheral hearing.

Audiologist — An individual trained in the identification and rehabilitative management of hearing disorders. Individual must possess at a minimum a master's degree in Audiology and meet the requirements of the American Speech, Language and Hearing Association for certification to practice. (Individual states may require licensure in addition to the above requirements.)

AUDIOMETRY	The measurement of hearing.
AURICLE	The external ear, also referred to as pinna. This structure acts to accept and funnel sound to the middle ear.
AUTISM	A condition first described by Leo Kanner. It is characterized by aloofness, lack of relatedness, and most often muteness. These symptoms begin during the first three years of life. Current interventions do not seem to have much impact, nor do they seem to ameliorate this condition.
BABBLING	Sounds that infants produce at approximately three months of age.
BEHAVIORAL TESTING	Observation of infants behavior in response to various auditory-test stimuli.
BONE CONDUCTION	Measurement made with an oscillator behind the ear on the mastoid bone that evaluates the hearing sensitivity of the inner ear.
BRAINSTEM	The area that links the peripheral hearing mechanism to the brain (cortex).
CENTRAL AUDITORY NERVOUS SYSTEM	The complicated pathways leading from the VIII Nerve (Auditory Nerve) to the brain. This system encompasses the brainstem and cortical regions of the brain.
CENTRAL AUDITORY PROCESSING DISORDER (CAP)	Problems in deciphering and understanding verbal messages.
COCHLEA	Snail-shaped structure also referred to as the inner ear. This structure contains the essential end organ for hearing.

Cochlear Nucleus	Located in the brainstem and thought to be the initial stage in the processing of sound.
Cognitive Development	The stage-by-stage development, as conceptualized by Jean Piaget of remembering, reasoning, and logical thinking.
Communication	System of sending, understanding and formulating a specific signal to send or exchange information.
Conductive Hearing Loss	Hearing loss occurring in the outer or middle ear and affecting the conduction of sound through to the cochlea or inner ear.
Cortex	The topmost layer of the brain often referred to as the gray matter.
Cylert	Prescription medication often used for ADHD.
Dyslexia	A learning problem that manifests itself in a deficit in reading skills.
Ego-Centricity	Belief that all people think the same thoughts at the same time as one another.
Encoding	Process of converting an idea into an audible or visual signal.
Eustachian Tube	A tubelike structure stretching from the nasopharynx to the middle-ear cavity. The function of this tube is to equalize pressure within the head by bringing air into the middle-ear space.
Frequency	The highness or lowness of a sound measured in hertz (Hz) or (cps) cycles per second. Pitch is the psychological correlate of frequency.

Functional Integrity	The ability of one's hearing system, both peripheral and central, to receive and process information.
Herschl's Gyrus	Located in the temporal lobe of the brain. This is thought to be the end point of the auditory pathway.
Immittance/Impedance	A procedure used to obtain further information regarding the stability of the middle-ear system.
Incus	A tiny bone in the middle ear, also referred to as the hammer because of its resemblance to that object. The incus attaches to the malleus on one end and medially to the stapes.
Inflection	A change in intonation patterns during speech.
Intensity	The loudness or softness of a sound measured in decibels (dB).
Irreversibility	The inability of children to retrace their thinking from their conclusions to their original premises.
Language	An arbitrary system for concept representation. Symbols that are gestural, pictorial, or verbal may be used. A mutually understood set of rules is associated.
Language Disability	A problem in one or more areas of language; i.e., pragmatics, semantics, etc.
Linguistic Competence	A speaker's knowledge of the system and rules for understanding and sending messages through language.

Lobe — One of four areas of the brain: occipital, parietal, temporal and frontal.

Malleus — A tiny bone in the middle ear, also referred to as the hammer because of its resemblance to that object. The malleus attaches to the tympanic membrane on one end and to the incus medially.

Medulla — The lowest portion of the brain, connecting the pons with the spinal cord.

Minimal Brain Dysfunction — Neurological deficits as evidenced by some impairment in motor skills and learning. The impairments may be subtle.

Morphology — An area of language that refers to rules regarding changes in meaning among words within an utterance.

Nasopharynx — The area where the back of the nose and throat connect.

Occipital Lobe — Area of brain where visual processing occurs.

Ossicle — Three tiny bones called the malleus, incus, and stapes, located behind the tympanic membrane in the middle ear.

Perceptual — Focusing of visual attention on an object and coming to an understanding of the object based on its visual characteristics.

Peripheral Hearing Mechanism — The structures of the ear responsible for receiving sound (outer ear), conducting sound (middle ear), and initially analyzing it (inner ear), before it is sent to brain for storage and analysis.

PHONATE	Production of a sound as a result of a vibration of vocal folds.
PHONEMES	The smallest unit of sound that is responsible for changing meaning.
PHONOLOGY	An area of language that includes specified rules involving speech sounds and patterns of speech.
PRAGMATICS	Area of language associated with communication intent and content.
PRECONCEPTUAL	Arises from stage of preoperational thought when children assume that evidence is incorrect if it contradicts their ideas.
PREOPERATIONAL	Stage of cognitive development, described by Piaget, and characterized by a visual understanding of events and experiences.
PRE-SPEECH	The sounds and intonation patterns infants produce before meaningful utterances are produced.
REPRESENTATIONS	The ability to form pictures of nonpresent objects in one's head.
RITALIN	Prescription medication used to suppress symptoms of ADHD.
SEMANTICS	An area of language that involves meaning of words.
SENSORINEURAL HEARING LOSS	Hearing loss occurring in the cochlea or the neural structures that lie beyond. A loss in this area causes a decrease in the intensity of sound as well as sound distortion.

Serous Otitus Media	An inflammation of the middle ear that causes fluid to accumulate.
Specific Learning Disability	A deficit in learning that can be identified. For example: A disability in processing sound, a disability in word recognition, a disability in short-term memory, etc.
Speech	A process in which the oral motor structures, governed by the neuro system produces sound. Speech is a verbal means of communication.
Speech Audiometric Testing	A procedure used to determine the impact of hearing loss on a person's understanding of speech.
Stapes	A tiny bone in the middle ear, also referred to as the stirrup because of its resemblance to that object. The stapes attaches to the incus on one end and to the inner ear or cochlea medially.
Symbolism	A sign that stands for an object; E.g., the word *apple* stands for the object.
Symbols	Something that stands for, represents, or suggests another thing.
Syntax	An area of language that is concerned with word order.
Tympanic Membrane	An elastic structure located at the end of the ear canal also referred to as the ear drum.
Vestibular System	Three semicircular canals that connect to the cochlea and are responsible for balance.

VIII Cranial Nerve (Eighth Nerve) This structure, also referred to as the auditory nerve, carries electrical impulses from the inner ear (cochlea) and the vestibular system (semicircular canals) to the brain.

Vocal Play Sounds that an infant produces at approximately six months of age consisting of consonants and vowel combinations. For example: "ma," "da," "ba."

______Lucy Freeman
OUR INNER WORLD OF RAGE
Understanding and Transforming the Power of Anger
A psychoanalytic examination of the anger that burns within us and which can be used to save or slowly destroy us. Sheds light on all expressions of rage, from the murderer to the suicide to those of us who feel depressed and angry but are unaware of the real cause.
$9.95 paperback

____John Gerdtz and Joel Bregman, M. D.
AUTISM
A Practical Guide for Those Who Help Others
An up-to-date and comprehensive guidebook for everyone who works with autistic children, adolescents, adults, and their families. Includes latest information on medications. $17.95

_____Marion Howard
HOW TO HELP YOUR TEENAGER
POSTPONE SEXUAL INVOLVEMENT
Based on a national educational program that works, this book advises parents, teachers, and counselors on how they can help their teens resist social and peer pressures regarding sex. $9.95 paperback

_____Marion Howard
SOMETIMES I WONDER ABOUT ME
Teenagers and Mental Health
Combines fictional narratives with sound, understandable professional advice to help teenagers recognize the difference between serious problems and normal problems of adjustment. $9.95 paperback

_____Charles H. Huber and Barbara A. Backlund
THE TWENTY MINUTE COUNSELOR
Transforming Brief Conversations into Effective Helping Experiences
Expert advice for anyone who by necessity must often counsel "on the run" or in a short period of time. $16.95

_____E. Clay Jorgensen
CHILD ABUSE
A Practical Guide for Those Who Help Others
Essential information and practical advice for caregivers called upon to help both child and parent in child abuse. $16.95

_____Eugene Kennedy
CRISIS COUNSELING
The Essential Guide for Nonprofessional Counselors
"An outstanding author of books on personal growth selects types of personal crises that our present life-style has made commonplace and suggests effective ways to deal with them."—*Best Sellers* $10.95

_____Eugene Kennedy and Sara Charles, M. D.
ON BECOMING A COUNSELOR
A Basic Guide for Nonprofessional Counselors
New expanded edition of an indispensable resource. A patient-oriented, clinically directed field guide to understanding and responding to troubled people. $27.95 hardcover
$15.95 paperback

_____Eugene Kennedy
SEXUAL COUNSELING
A Practical Guide for Those Who Help Others
Newly revised and up-to-date edition, with a new chapter on the counselor and AIDS, of an essential book on counseling people with sexual problems. $17.95

_____Bonnie Lester
WOMEN AND AIDS
A Practical Guide for Those Who Help Others
Provides positive ways for women to deal with their fears, and to help others who react with fear to people who have AIDS. $15.95

_____Robert J. Lovinger
RELIGION AND COUNSELING
The Psychological Impact of Religious Belief
How counselors and clergy can best understand the important emotional significance of religious thoughts and feelings. $17.95

_____ Sophie L. Lovinger, Mary Ellen Brandell, and
Linda Seestedt-Stanford
LANGUAGE LEARNING DISABILITIES
A New and Practical Approach for Those Who Work with Children and Their Families
Here is new information, together with practical suggestions, on how teachers, therapists, and families can work together to give learning disabled children new strengths. $22.95

_____ Helen B. McDonald and Audrey I. Steinhorn
HOMOSEXUALITY
A Practical Guide to Counseling Lesbians, Gay Men, and Their Families
A sensitive guide to better understanding and counseling gays, lesbians, and their parents, at every stage of their lives. $17.95

_____ James McGuirk and Mary Elizabeth McGuirk
FOR WANT OF A CHILD
A Psychologist and His Wife Explore the Emotional Effects and Challenges of Infertility
A new understanding of infertility that comes from one couple's lived experience, as well as sound professional advice for couples and counselors. $17.95

_____ Janice N. McLean and Sheila A. Knights
PHOBICS AND OTHER PANIC VICTIMS
A Practical Guide for Those Who Help Them
"A must for the phobic, spouse and family, and for the physician and support people who help them." — Arthur B. Hardy, M. D., Founder, TERRAP Phobia Program $17.95

_____ John B. Mordock and William Van Ornum
CRISIS COUNSELING WITH CHILDREN AND ADOLESCENTS
A Guide for Nonprofessional Counselors
New Expanded Edition
"Every parent should keep this book on the shelf right next to the nutrition, medical, and Dr. Spock books."—*Marriage & Family Living*
$12.95

_____ John B. Mordock
COUNSELING CHILDREN
Basic Principles for Helping the Troubled and Defiant Child
Helps counselors consider the best route for a particular child, and offers proven principles and methods to counsel troubled children in a variety of situations. $17.95

_____Cherry Boone O'Neill
DEAR CHERRY
Questions and Answers on Eating Disorders
Practical and inspiring advice on eating disorders from the best- selling author of *Starving for Attention.* $8.95 paperback

_____Paul G. Quinnett
ON BECOMING A HEALTH
AND HUMAN SERVICES MANAGER
A Practical Guide for Clinicians and Counselors
A new and essential guide to management for everyone in the helping professions—from mental health to nursing, from social work to teaching. $19.95

_____Paul G. Quinnett
SUICIDE: THE FOREVER DECISION
For Those Thinking About Suicide,
and For Those Who Know, Love, or Counsel Them
"A treasure— this book can help save lives."—William Van Ornum, psychotherapist and author $18.95 hardcover $8.95 paperback

_____Paul G. Quinnett
WHEN SELF-HELP FAILS
A Consumer's Guide to Counseling Services
A guide to professional therapie. "Without a doubt one of the most honest, reassuring, nonpaternalistic, and useful self-help books ever to appear."—*Booklist* $10.95

_____Judah L. Ronch
ALZHEIMER'S DISEASE
A Practical Guide for Families and Other Caregivers
Must reading for everyone who must deal with the effects of this tragic disease on a daily basis. Filled with examples as well as facts, this book provides insights into dealing with one's feelings as well as with such practical advice as how to choose long-term care. $11.95 paperback

_____Theodore Isaac Rubin, M. D.
ANTI-SEMITISM: A DISEASE OF THE MIND
"A most poignant and lucid psychological examination of a severe emotional disease. Dr. Rubin offers hope and understanding to the victim and to the bigot. A splendid job!"—Dr. Herbert S. Strean $14.95

_____Theodore Isaac Rubin, M.D.
CHILD POTENTIAL
Fulfilling Your Child's Intellectual, Emotional, and Creative Promise
Information, guidance, and wisdom—a treasury of fresh ideas for parents to help their children become their best selves.
$18.95 hardcover $11.95 paperback

_____John R. Shack
COUPLES COUNSELING
A Practical Guide for Those Who Help Others
An essential guide to dealing with the 20 percent of all counseling situations that involve the relationship of two people. $17.95

_____Herbert S. Strean as told to Lucy Freeman
BEHIND THE COUCH
Revelations of a Psychoanalyst
"An entertaining account of an analyst's thoughts and feelings during the course of therapy."—*Psychology Today*
$11.95 paperback

_____Stuart Sutherland
THE INTERNATIONAL DICTIONARY OF PSYCHOLOGY
This new dictionary of psychology also covers a wide range of related disciplines, from anthropology to sociology. $49.95

_____Joan Leslie Taylor
IN THE LIGHT OF DYING
The Journals of a Hospice Volunteer
"Beautifully recounts the healing (our own) that results from service to others, and might well be considered as required reading for hospice volunteers." —Stephen Levine, author of *Who Dies?* $17.95